# Home Care i10 Cheat Sheet

## For fast icd-10 Coding
## In HHC with Adult Population
## Updated for Fiscal Year 2023
## Oct 1, 2022 thru Sep 30, 2023

GLB Worldwide
Kaneohe Hi

Home Care i10 Cheat Sheet



Library of Congress Control Number: 2017914763

Published by GLB Worldwide (Great Little Books), Kaneohe Hi

http://www.icd10cheatsheet.com

## Using This Cheat Sheet

Any Cheat Sheets is intended to help you accomplish tasks by providing needed information in a quick and easy format. This Cheat Sheet will shave considerable time off your i10 coding, usually 25% or more., and make it easier, too.

This Cheat Sheet is designed so it is easy to use by anyone who can read and use a dictionary.

The Main section is a simple alpha listing, like a dictionary. Each main entry is in bold letters. The i10 code is set off to the left. If there are variations, they are listed below the first entry. For example, leg cramps is a main entry with the code off-set to the left. Below it are variations: sleep related, Charley-horse, and carpo-pedal spasm.

Where it seems to make most sense, codes are listed by anatomical site. For example, a patient may have both a hip pressure ulcer and hip bursitis. You can find both codes quickly within a few entries of one another under HIP.

If a diagnosis has its own specific nomenclature, look there. This would be diagnoses like Legionnaires' disease or mumps. If there are multiple variations, they are listed, too.

In many cases, if other codes often accompany that main code, they are listed and identified as RELATED. For example, RELATED Anemia in chronic kidney disease is listed beneath CRD: chronic renal disease NOS and the codes for its various stages.

Related codes are not always needed. They are provided to save your time when they are required. If RELATED codes are not applicable, just ignore them.

Hundreds of 'abbreviated' diagnoses are coded. If source documents list an acronym you are unfamiliar with there is a good chance you won't need to look up the definition first. Look up the acronym in the Cheat Sheet and get the definition and codes in one search. Examples: ACD: adult celiac disease, EMF: endomyocardial fibrosis, PML: progressive multifocal leukoencephalopathy.

The codes provided in The i10 Cheat Sheet are best used with an adult population. There are no OB or Neo codes.

The Tables section includes groups of codes that often have so many variations that a table is the best way to include the most information. Take a few minutes to familiarize yourself with available tables. These can really save time!

Like anything, the more you use the Cheat Sheet the easier it gets and the faster you will code. Like any cheat sheet, this is an abridged version of a larger reference - published by the Centers for Medicare and Medicaid.

There is ample room for you to add notes. If you find that a code you use often is not listed, write it in. It will make YOUR cheat sheet even more effective for you. I published the icd-9 Cheat Sheet for 23 years and it got better every year because coders shared. Besides new codes from CMS, each yearly edition contained "new" codes from coders. If you make notes, feel free to share. Send your code ideas to info@glbworld.com

When I coded records for home health, I made a cheat sheet that was always evolving. When I began the day, I usually had a sizeable stack of records to start with and more were added throughout the day. I always went through and coded with my cheat sheet first. Often, nothing more was needed. Then I used the full code text from CMS (free online) to finish the others. I routinely coded many more records than the other coders.

Then one fateful day, something wonderful happened. Another coder asked if she could make a copy of my cheat sheet to use. Of course! An idea was born and we all coded happily ever after - at least until the company was sold.

# A

**E7081** **AADC: Aromatic L-amino acid decarboxylase Deficiency**

**R100** **Abdomen acute**

**K660** **Abdomen adhesions postinfection / postop NOS**
postinfection / postop w/obstruction K565

**S346xx-** **Abdomen peripheral nerve injury**
7th character indicates encounter
A- initial encounter D- subsequent encounter S- sequela

**I714** **Abdominal aneurysm aorta**
w/ rupture I713

**K551** **Abdominal angina**

**M79A3** **Abdominal compartment syndrome nontraumatic**

**T79A3X -** **Abdominal compartment syndrome traumatic**
7th character indicates encounter (trauma only)
A-initial encounter D-subsequent encounter S-sequela

**R109** **Abdominal cramps NOS**

**R140** **Abdominal distension**

**K632** **Abdominal fistula (wall)**

**R188** **Abdominal fluid accumulation NOS**

**K469** **Abdominal hernia NOS**
w/gangrene K461 w/obstruction K460
ventral incisional/postop NOS K432 w/gangrene K431
ventral NOS K439

**R1084** **Abdominal pain generalized NOS**

**R1030** **Abdominal pain local lower NOS**
RLQ R1031 LLQ R1032 Periumbilical R1033

**R1010** **Abdominal pain local upper NOS**
RUQ R1011 LUQ R1012 epigastric R1013

**R1930** **Abdominal rigidity NOS**
RUQ R1931 LUQ R1932
RLQ R1933 LLQ R1934
periumbilic R1935 epigastric R1936
generalized R1937

**R1900** **Abdominal swelling, mass, lump NOS**
RUQ R1901 LUQ R1902
RLQ R1903 LLQ R1904
Periumbilic R1905 Epigastric R1906
Generalized R1907 Other R1909

**R10819** **Abdominal tenderness NOS**

RUQ R10811 LUQ R10812
RLQ R10813 LLQ R10814
periumbilic R10815 epigastric R10816 generalized R10817

**R10829** **Abdominal tenderness REBOUND NOS**

RUQ R10821 LUQ R10822
RLQ R10823 LLQ R10824
periumbilic R10825 epigastric R10826 generalized R10827

**L02211** **Abdominal wall abscess cutaneous, code organism if known**

**L02231** **Abdominal wall carbuncle, code organism if known**

**K632** **Abdominal wall fistula NOS**

**L02221** **Abdominal wall furuncle/boil, code organism if known**

**I330** **ABE: acute bacterial endocarditis**

**L0390** **Abscess NOS**

**F558** **Abuse of non-psychoactive substances other**

antacids F550 herbal / folk remedies F551
laxative F552 steroids / hormones F553 vitamins F554

**B889** **Acariasis NOS**

**K900** **ACD: adult celiac disease**

Code also exocrine pancreatic insufficiency K8681
RELATED Dermatitis herpetiformis L130 gluten ataxia G3281

**S32436 -** **Acetabulum fracture column anterior [iliopubic] Nondisplaced unspecified**

Nondisplaced right S32434- l eft S32435-
Displaced: right S32431- l eft S32432- unspecified S32433-
Posterior column [ilioischial] = change 5th character to 4
Add the appropriate 7th character:
initial encounter: closed fracture = A open fracture = B
subsequent encounter: routine healing = D delayed healing = G
subsequent encounter fracture w/ nonunion = K sequela = S

**S32456 -** **Acetabulum fracture transverse Nondisplaced unspecified**

Nondisplaced right S32454- left S32455-
Displaced: right S32451- left S32452- unspecified S32453-
Associated transverse-posterior = change 5th character to 6
Dome fracture = change 5th character to 8
Other specified fracture: right S32491- left S32492- unspecified S32499-
Add the appropriate 7th character:
initial encounter: closed fracture = A open fracture = B
subsequent encounter: routine healing = D delayed healing = G
subsequent encounter fracture w/ nonunion = K sequela = S

**S32409 -** **Acetabulum fracture Unspecified NOS**

right ilium S32401- left ilium S32402
Add the appropriate 7th character:
initial encounter: closed fracture = A open fracture = B
subsequent encounter: routine healing = D delayed healing = G
subsequent encounter fracture w/ nonunion = K sequela = S

**S32416 -** **Acetabulum fracture wall anterior Nondisplaced unspecified**

Nondisplaced right S32414- left S32415
Displaced: right S32411- left S32412- unspecified S32413-
Posterior wall = change 5th character to 2
Medial wall = change 5th character to 7
Add the appropriate 7th character:
initial encounter: closed fracture = A open fracture = B
subsequent encounter: routine healing = D delayed healing = G
subsequent encounter fracture w/ nonunion = K sequela = S

**R824** **Acetonuria**

**K220** **Achalasia NOS / cardia / esophageal**

**M7660** **Achilles tendinitis unspecified**

right M7661 left M7662

**K3183** **Achlorhydria**

**E8720** **Acidosis lactic/metabolic/NOS**

lactic/metabolic Acute E8721
lactic/metabolic Chronic E8722
Other / Respiratory NOS E8729
renal / kidney tubular N2589

**G803** **ACP: athetoid cerebral palsy**

**K59.81** **ACPO: Acute colonic pseudo-obstruction**

**S43109-** **Acromioclavicular joint dislocation unspecified**

right S43101- left S43102-
7th character indicates encounter
A - initial encounter D - subsequent encounter S - sequela

**S4350x -** **Acromioclavicular sprain unspecified**

right S4361x- left S4362x
7th character indicates encounter
A -initial encounter D -subsequent encounter S -sequela

**M5382** **ACS: acute cervical spine syndrome**

**A429** **Actinomycosis NOS**

Pulmonary A420 sepsis A427 abdominal A421
Cervicofacial A422 meningitis A4281 encephalitis A4282
Other forms A4289
RELATED cystitis N3080 w/ hematuria N3081
RELATED meningitis G01 RELATED prostatitis N51

**F909** **ADD: attention deficit disorder NOS**

predominantly inattentive F900 predominantly hyperactive F901
combined type F902 other F908

**E271** **Addison's disease primary (adrenocortical insufficiency)**

crisis E272 NOS E2740
drug induced E273 tuberculous A187
RELATED Addison's anemia D510

**G0400** **ADEM: acute disseminated encephalitis and encephalomyelitis NOS**

postinfectious G0401 postimmunization G0402 noninfectious G0481

**Adenitis - SEE Lymphadenitis**

**J3503** **Adenoiditis & tonsillitis chronic**

adenoiditis alone chronic J3502

**D8130** **Adenosine deaminase deficiency, unspecified, NOS**

Severe combined immunodeficiency due to, D8131 (ADA deficiency with SCID)
Adenosine deaminase 2 deficiency D8132 (ADA2 deficiency, ADA deficiency type 2)
(ADA2 deficiency, ADA deficiency type 2)

**ADHD: SEE ADD**

**E342** **ADHES: antidiuretic hormone secretion ectopic (ADH)**

**E222** **ADHIS: antidiuretic hormone secretion inappropriate (SIADH)**

**T50905-** **ADR: adverse drug reaction, unspecified drug**

penicillins T360x5- tetracyclines T365x5-
sulfonamide T370x5- insulin & oral antidiabetics T383x5-
aspirin T39015- other salicylates T39095-
other NSAIDS T39395- barbiturates T423x5-
antiallergic/antiemetic T450x5- antineoplastic T451x5-
thrombolytic T45615- hemostatic T45625-
coronary vasodilator T463x5- antivaricose T468x5-
multiple drugs T50915- (code also specific drugs)
7th character indicates encounter:
A- initial encounter D- subsequent encounter S- sequela

**Adrenal hyperplasia SEE Cushing's Syndrome**

**E259** **Adrenogenital syndrome NOS**

**Z48815** **Aftercare digestive system postop**

**Z5189** **Aftercare NOS (SEE specific type also, eg wound, colostomy)**

NEC Z5189 tracheostomy Z430
postop drain: change or remove Z4803

**Z483** **Aftercare oncology surgery**

**Z471** **Aftercare orthopedic following joint replacement re-surgery**

Z472 following removal of internal fixation device
Z4733 following explantation of knee joint prosthesis
Z4732 following explantation of hip joint prosthesis
Z4731 following explantation of shoulder joint prosthesis
Z4782 following scoliosis surgery Z4789 other orthopedic aftercare
Z4781 following surgical amputation
RELATED AMPUTATIONS hand: rt Z89111 lt Z89112 unsp Z89119
arm rt Z89119 lt Z89202 unsp Z89209
below elbow rt Z89519 lt Z89212 unsp Z89219
leg rt Z89611 lt Z89612 unsp Z89619
below knee rt Z89619 lt Z89512 unsp Z89519

**Z471** **Aftercare Postop orthopedic joint replacement**

Use additional code below to identify the joint
shoulder: right Z96611 left Z96612 unsp Z96619
elbow: right Z96621 left Z96622 unsp Z96629
wrist: right Z96631 left Z96632 unsp Z96639
hip: right Z96641 left Z96642 bilat Z96643 unsp Z96649
knee: right Z96651 left Z96652 bilat Z96653 unsp Z96659
ankle: right Z96661 left Z96662 unsp Z96669
finger: right Z96691 left Z96692 bilat Z96693
other Z96698

**Z435** **Aftercare urinary artificial opening cystostomy**

other Z436

**N009** **AGN: acute glomerulonephritis**

**D66** **AHGD: antihemophilic globulin deficiency**

**T80310-** **AHTR: acute hemolytic transfusion reaction d/t ABO incompatibility within 24 hrs of**

d/t Rh incompatibility T80410-
7th character indicates encounter
A- initial encounter D- subsequent encounter S- sequela

**AICD complication**

mechanical breakdown T82518- displacement T82528-
leakage T82538- Infection T827xx-
7th character indicates encounter
A- initial encounter D- subsequent encounter S- sequela

**Z4502** **AICD fitting & adjustment**

**Z95810** **AICD status**

**Z717** **Aids counseling**

**R75** **Aids HIV lab evidence inconclusive**

**Z21** **Aids infection asymptomatic status / HIV positive NOS**

**B20** **AIDS: acquired immunodeficiency syndrome**

RELATED Kaposi's sarcomas:
gastrointestinal organ C464 palate (hard) (soft) C462
rectum C464 lymph node(s) C463
ung: unsp C4650 right C4651 left C4652
lung: unsp C4650 right C4651 left C4652

**K6282** **AIN: anal intraepithelial neoplasia (histologically confirmed) NOS/grade I /grade II**

grade III, severe D013

**E8021** **AIP: acute intermittent porphyria**

**T800XX-** **Air embolism following infusion, transfusion and therapeutic injection**

7th character indicates encounter
A- initial encounter D- subsequent encounter S- sequela

**G2571** **Akathisia Drug induced**

**N179** **AKF: acute kidney failure NOS nontraumatic**

w/tubular necrosis N170 w/acute cortical necrosis N171
w/medullary necrosis N172 other spec N178

**F1010** **Alcohol abuse uncomplicated**

w/intoxication: uncomplicated F10120
delirium F10121 unspecified F10129
alcohol induced psychosis w/ delusions F10150
alcohol hallucinations F10151 unsp F10159
alcohol induced: anxiety F10180 sexual dysfunction F10181
alcohol induced: sleep disorder F10182 other disorder F10188
alcohol induced mood disorder F1014
abuse w/unsp disorder F1019
in remission F1011

**F10139** **Alcohol abuse with withdrawal unspecified**

Alcohol abuse with withdrawal, uncomplicated F10130
Alcohol abuse with withdrawal delirium F10131
Alcohol abuse w/ withdrawal w/ perceptual disturbance F10132

**F10939** **Alcohol use, unspecified with withdrawal, unspecified**

Alcohol use, unspecified with withdrawal, uncomplicated F10930
Alcohol use, unspecified with withdrawal delirium F10931
Alcohol use, unspecified with withdrawal with perceptual disturbance F10932

**F10231** **Alcohol withdrawal delirium**

**F10239** **Alcohol withdrawal syndrome/psychosis NOS**

**Z6372** **Alcoholism in family**

**F1020** **Alcoholism NOS**

in remission F1021
w/mood disorder F1024
w/persisting dementia F1027

**E269** **Aldosteronism NOS (also hyperaldosteronism)**

other primary E2609 Secondary E261
Bartler's E2681 Conn's syndrome E2601
glucocorticoid-remediable E2602

**R29898** **ALF: acute loss of function**

**E873** **Alkalosis NOS**

**C9100** **ALL: acute lymphoid leukemia NOS**

in remission C9101 in relapse C9102

**Z880** **Allergy penicillin**

**Z91013** **Allergy seafood**

**G3181** **Alpers disease**

**D8982** **ALPS: autoimmune lymphoproliferative syndrome**

**G1221** **ALS: amyotrophic lateral sclerosis**

**G309** **Alzheimer's NOS Do not use with senile codes**

early onset G300 late onset G301 other G308
RELATED dementia w/behavioral disturbance F0281
RELATED dementia w/o behavioral disturbance F0280
RELATED delerium F05

**R262** **Ambulation difficulty NOS**

ataxic gait R260 paralytic gait R261
unsteady on feet R2681 other specified R2689
unspecified gait difficulty R269

**AMD: age related macular degenertion SEE ARMD**

**A069** **Amebiasis NOS**

acute dysentery A060 chronic intestinal A061
nondysenteric colitis A062 Ameboma A063
hepatic A064 lung abscess (or lung w/liver) A065
brain abscess A066 Cutaneous A067
cystitis A0681 Other genitourinary A0682
other A0689

**R3121** **AMH: Asymptomatic microscopic hematuria**

**I213** **AMI: acute myocardial infarction NOS**

RELATED
exposure to environmental tobacco smoke Z7722
history of tobacco dependence Z87891
occupational exposure to environmental tobacco smoke Z5731
Nicotine dependence NOS F17209 SEE Nicotine dependence for more
tobacco use Z720

**I21A1** **AMI: acute myocardial infarction type 2 -- Code underlying cause first**

**A319** **AMI: atypical mycobacterial infection NOS**

cutaneous A311 pulmonary A310

**C9200** **AML: acute myeloid leukemia NOS**

in remission C9201 in relapse C9202

**R413** **Amnesia NOS**

anterograde R411 retrograde R412

**E859** **Amyloidosis unspecified**

non-neuropathic E850 neuropathic E851
heredofamilial E852
secondary systemic / hemodialysis associated E853
localized / organ limited E854
other NEC E8589 light chain E8581
senile systemic/Wild-type transthyretin-related (ATTR) E8582

**I7782** **ANCA: Antineutrophilic cytoplasmic antibody vasculitis**

**E3450** **Androgen sensitivity syndrome NOS**

complete E3451 partial E3452

**D5529** **Anemia d/t other disorders of glycolytic enzymes**

Includes Hexokinase deficiency anemia
and Triose-phosphate isomerase deficiency anemia

**D5521** **Anemia d/t pyruvate kinase deficiency**

**D519** **Anemia deficiency B12 NOS**

d/t intrinsic factor deficiency D510
d/t selective malabsorption D511
other dietary deficiency D513
other D518
transcobalamin II deficiency D512

**D529** **Anemia deficiency folate NOS**

dietary deficiency D520 drug-induced D521
other D528

**D509** **Anemia deficiency iron NOS**

secondary to blood loss D500
secondary to inadequate intake D508
sideropenic dysphagia D501

**D530** **Anemia deficiency protein**

**D6481** **Anemia due to antineoplastic chemotherapy**

RELATED
anemia in neoplastic disease D630
aplastic anemia due to antineoplastic chemotherapy D611

**D631** **Anemia due to chronic kidney disease**

Code first underlying chronic kidney disease

**D630** **Anemia due to neoplastic disease - Code first neoplasm**

RELATED anemia due to antineoplastic chemotherapy D6481

**D599** **Anemia hemolytic acquired NOS**

nonautoimmune: drug induced D592 other D594
hemolytic-uremic syndrome NOS D5930
hemolytic-uremic syndrome infection associated D5931
hemolytic-uremic syndrome hereditary D5932
hemolytic-uremic syndrome other D5939
other hemolytic anemia D598

**D5910** **Anemia hemolytic autoimmune unspecified**

Drug-induced D590
Warm D5911 Cold D5912 Mixed D5913
Other autoimmune hemolytic anemia D5919

**D539** **Anemia nutritional NOS / simple chronic**

scorbutic D532 protein D530
other nutritional D538 galoblastic NOS D531

**D62** **Anemia posthemorrhagic acute**

d/t chronic blood loss D500

**D464** **Anemia refractory unspecified**

with ring sideroblasts (RARS) D461
with excess of blasts, unspecified (RAEB NOS) D4620
with excess of blasts 1 (RAEB 1) D4621
with excess of blasts 2 (RAEB 2) D4622
without ring sideroblasts, so stated D460

**D649** **Anemia unspecified**

**D513** **Anemia vegan**

**I209** **Angina pectoris NOS**

unstable I200 postinfarction I237 other I208
w/documented spasm I201 Refractory I202
RELATED
exposure to environmental tobacco smoke Z7722
history of tobacco dependence Z87891
occupational exposure to environmental tobacco smoke Z5731
Nicotine dependence NOS F17209 SEE Nicotine dependence for more
tobacco use Z720

**G0430** **ANHE: acute necrotizing hemorrhagic encephalopathy NOS**

postinfectious G0431 postimmunization G0432 other G0439

**L02429** **Ankle boil / furuncle unspecified**

right L02425 left L02426

**M71479** **Ankle calcification unspecified**

right M71471 left M71472

**L02439** **Ankle carbuncle unspecified**

right L02435 left L02436

**M9279** **Ankle chondromalacia unspecified**

right M94271 left M94272

**M24573** **Ankle contractures unspecified**

right M24571 left M24572

**M25473** **Ankle effusion unspecified**

right M25471 left M25472

**M7750** **Ankle enthesopathy unspecified ankle (also foot)**

Right M7751 left M7752

**M84473 -** **Ankle fracture pathological NOS unspecified Change 4th character to 5 for 'in neop**

right M84471- left M84472-
7th character indicates encounter/status
A - initial S - sequela
D - subsequent routine healing
G - subsequent delayed healing
K - subsequent nonunion P - subsequent malunion

**M25073** **Ankle hemarthrosis unspecified**

right M25071 left M25072

**M24873** **Ankle instability NOS unspecified**

right M24871 left M24872

**M24073** **Ankle joint mice unspecified**

right M24071 left M24072

**Ankle osteomyelitis**

acute hematogenous: unsp M86079 right M86071 left M86072
other acute: unsp M86179 right M86171 left M86172
subacute: unsp M86279 right M86271 left M86272
chronic multifocal: unsp M86379 right M86371 left M86372
chronic, draining sinus: unsp M86479 right M86471 left 86472
chronic hematogenous: unsp M86579 right M86571 left M86572
other chronic: unsp M86679 right M86671 left M86672

**M80079-** **Ankle osteoporosis age related w/current fracture unspecified**

right M80071- left M80072 -
7th character indicates encounter/status
A- initia l D- subsequent routine healing
G- subsequent delayed healing S- sequela
K- subsequent nonunion P- subsequent malunion

**Z96669** **Ankle replacement status unspecified**

right Z96661 left Z96662

**M25673** **Ankle stiffness (joint) NOS unspecified**

right M25671 left M25672

**Ankle swelling (joint) SEE ankle effusion**

**L97329** **Ankle ulcer non-pressure chronic LEFT NOS**

limited to skin L97321 w/fat layer exposed L97322
w/muscle necrosis L97323 w/bone necrosis L97324
w/muscle involvement without necrosis L97325
w/bone involvement without necrosis L97326
w/ other specified severity L97328
These codes also for midfoot
RIGHT SIDE Change character five to 1
UNSPECIFIED SIDE Change character five to 0

**L89529** **Ankle ulcer pressure left NOS**

unstageable L89520
stage 1 L89521 stage 2 L89522
stage 3 L89523 stage 4 L89524
pressure-induced deep tissue damage L89526
RIGHT SIDE change character five to 1
UNSPECIFIED SIDE change character five to 0

**Anogenital herpes SEE Herpes simplex Anogenital**

**K612** **Anorectal abscess / cellulitis**

**K605** **Anorectal fistula**

**K615** **Anorectal region Supralevator abscess**

**F5000** **Anorexia nervosa NOS**

restricting type F5001 binge eating/purging type F5002

**R630** **Anorexia NOS (simple, loss of appetite)**

**K8591** **ANP: acute necrotizing pancreatitis, unspecified type NOS**

unspecified type: infected K8592
Idiopathic: NOS K8501 infected K8502
Biliary: NOS K8511 infected K8512
Alcohol induced: NOS K8521 infected K8522
Drug induced: NOS K8531 infected K8532
Other: NOS K8581 infected K8582
SEE Pancreatitis acute for w/o necrosis or infection

**I808** **Antecubital thrombophlebitis**

**G8382** **Anterior cord syndrome**

**A229** **Anthrax unspecified**

Cutaneous A220 Pulmonary A221
Gastrointestinal A222 Anthrax sepsis A227
Other A228

**D6832** **Anticoagulant induced hemorrhage**

**Z7901** **Anticoagulant use long term current - includes aftercare**

RELATED drug level monitoring Z5181

**A691** **ANUG: acute necrotizing ulcerative gingivitis**

**R34** **Anuria NOS**

postop N990 traumatic T795XX -
for traumatic code 7th character indicates encounter
A- initial encounter D- subsequent encounter S- sequela

**K610** **Anus abscess / cellulitis**

RELATED intrasphincteric abscess K614

**K6289** **Anus cyst NOS**

**K6282** **Anus dysplasia NOS**

**K602** **Anus fissure NOS**

acute K600 chronic K601

**K603** **Anus fistula**

**K6289** **Anus granuloma/ irritation NOS**

**K625** **Anus hemorrhage**

**A563** **Anus infection d/t chlamydia trachomatis**

**Anus neoplasm**

malignant unspecified C210  malignant canal C211
malignant cloacogenic zone  C212
malignant overlapping sites w/rectum C218
Secondary C785  Benign D129
Mets to bone C7951  mets to unsp lymph nodes C779
Mets to intraabdominal lymph node C772
Mets to intrapelvic lymph node C775

**K620** **Anus polyp**

**K622** **Anus prolapse**

**K624** **Anus stenosis/stricture**

**A1832** **Anus tuberculosis NOS**

**F419** **Anxiety NOS**

**I719** **Aorta aneurysm NOS**

NOS w/rupture I718

**I7110** **Aorta aneurysm ruptured unspecified**

Aorta aneurysm ruptured ascending I7111
Aorta aneurysm ruptured aortic arch I7112
Aorta aneurysm ruptured descending thoracic I7113

**I7120** **Aorta aneurysm without rupture unspecified**

Aorta aneurysm without rupture ascending I7121
Aorta aneurysm without rupture aortic arch I7122
Aorta aneurysm without rupture descending thoracic I7123

**I7100** **Aorta dissection NOS**

thoracic: ascending I71010 arch I71011 descending I71012 unspec I71019
abdominal I7102  thoracoabdominal I7103

**I7781** **Aorta ectasia**

**I7410** **Aorta embolism and thrombosis NOS**

abdominal saddle embolus I7401
abdominal other I7409
thoracic I7411  other I7419

**I7130** **Aortic abdominal aneurysm, ruptured unspecified**

Aortic abdominal aneurysm Pararenal, ruptured I7131
Aortic abdominal aneurysm Juxtarenal ruptured I7132
Aortic abdominal aneurysm Infrarenal ruptured I7133
Aortic abdominal aneurysm unspecified w/o rupture I7140
Aortic abdominal aneurysm Pararenal, w/o rupture I7141
Aortic abdominal aneurysm Juxtarenal w/o rupture I7142
Aortic abdominal aneurysm Infrarenal w/o rupture I7143

| | |
|---|---|
| **I7150** | **Aortic Thoracoabdominal aneurysm, ruptured unspecified** |
| | Aortic Thoracoabdominal aneurysm Supraceliac ruptured I7151<br>Aortic Thoracoabdominal aneurysm Paravisceral ruptured I7152<br>Aortic Thoracoabdominal aneurysm without rupture unspecified I7160<br>Aortic Thoracoabdominal aneurysm without rupture Supraceliac I7161<br>Aortic Thoracoabdominal aneurysm without rupture Paravisceral I7162 |
| **I359** | **Aortic valve disorder nonrheumatic unspecified** |
| | stenosis I350 insufficiency I351<br>stenosis w/insufficiency I352<br>other I358 |
| **T8201XA** | **Aortic valve prosthesis mechanical malfunction initial encounter** |
| | subsequent encounter T8201XD sequela T8201XS |
| **I351** | **Aortic valve regurgitation NOS** |
| | rheumatic I061 |
| **I062** | **Aortic valve rheumatic stenosis w/insufficiency** |
| | stenosis NOS I060 |
| **D8182** | **APDS: Activated Phosphoinositide 3-kinase Delta Syndrome** |
| | Code also, if applicable, any associated manifestations |
| **J810** | **APE: acute pulmonary edema** |
| **I2699** | **APE: acute pulmonary embolism NOS (w/o cor pulmonale)** |
| | Single subsegmental pulmonary embolism NOS I2693<br>Multiple subsegmental pulmonary embolism I2694 |
| **R130** | **Aphagia NOS** |
| | psychogenic F509 |
| **R4701** | **Aphasia ataxic/ Broca's/ expressive/ motor/ NOS/ sensory** |
| | specified as sequelae of CVA or CVD late effect I69920 |
| **Q612** | **APKD: adult type polycystic kidney disease congenital** |
| **C9240** | **APL: acute promyelocytic leukemia NOS** |
| | in remission C9241 in relapse C9242 |
| | **Apnea Sleep - SEE sleep apnea** |

**K37** **Appendicitis unspecified**

Acute w/generalized peritonitis NOS K3520
Acute w/generalized peritonitis w/ abscess K3521
Acute w/localized peritonitis NOS K3530
Acute w/localized peritonitis & gangrene w/o perforation K3531
Acute w/perforation & localized peritonitis w/o abscess K3532
Acute w/perforation & localized peritonitis w/abscess K3533
Acute appendicitis NOS K3580
Other acute w/o perforation or gangrene K35890
Other acute w/o perforation w/gangrene K35891
Other / Chronic / Recurrent K36

**N80549** **Appendix endometriosis NOS unspecified depth**

Superficial N80541 Deep N80542

**G039** **Arachnoiditis spinal NOS**

**B20** **ARC: aids related complex**

**J80** **ARDS: acute respiratory distress syndrome**

**N179** **ARF: acute renal failure NOS**

w/ acute cortical necrosis N171
w/ medullary necrosis N172
w/ tubular necrosis N170

**L02413** **Arm abscess cutaneous right, code organism if known**

left L02414

**I721** **Arm artery aneurysm**

**Arm bone cyst**

solitary humerus: unsp M85429 right M85421 left M85422
solitary forearm: unsp M85439 right M85431 left M85432
aneurysmal cyst: change 4th digit to 5
other cyst: change 4th digit to 6

**L02433** **Arm carbuncle right, code organism if known**

left L02434

**G5640** **Arm causalgia NOS**

right G5641 left G5642 bilateral G5643

**Arm compartment syndrome - Includes all sites from shoulder to fingers**

nontraumatic: right M79A11 left M79A12 unsp M79A19
traumatic: right T79A11- left T79A12- unsp T79A19-
For traumatic codes, 7th character indicates encounter
A- initial encounter D- subsequent encounter S- sequela

**I82629** **Arm deep vein thrombosis acute NOS**

right I82621 left I82622 bilateral I82623

**I82729** **Arm deep vein thrombosis chronic NOS**

right I82721 left I82722 bilateral I82723
personal history of deep vein thrombosis Z86718

**R600** **Arm edema pitting/dependent/NOS**

**Arm embolism/thrombosis venous**

deep: acute I82629 chronic I82729
superficial: acute I82619 chronic I82719
NOS: acute I82609 chronic I82709

**Arm fracture pathological NOS -- Change 4th character to 5 for 'in neoplastic disease**

humerus: unsp M84429- right M84421- left M84422-
ulna: right M84431- left M84432-
radius: right M84433- left M84434-
forearm: unspecified M84439-
7th character indicates encounter/status
A - initial S - sequela
D - subsequent routine healing
G - subsequent delayed healing
K - subsequent nonunion P - subsequent malunion

**L02423** **Arm furuncle/boil right**

left L02424

**R2230** **Arm lump/mass/swelling skin NOS**

right R2231 left R2232 bilat R2233

**G5690** **Arm mononeuropathy NOS**

right G5691 left G5692 bilateral G5693

**G8320** **Arm monoplegia NOS**

dominant side: right G8321 left G8322
nondominant: right G8323 left G8324

**Arm osteonecrosis - 4th character listed below for cause**

humerus: unsp M87-29 right M87-21 left M87-22
radius: unsp M87-33 right M87-31 left M87-32
ulna: unsp M87-36 right M87-34 left M87-35
shoulder: unsp M87-19 right M87-11 left M87-12
carpus: unsp M87-39 right M87-37 left M87-38
hand: unsp M87-43 right M87-41 left M87-42
finger: unsp M87-46 right M87-44 left M87-45
4th character cause =
idiopathic aseptic = 0 d/t drugs = 1 d/t trauma = 2
other secondary = 3 other = 8

**Arm osteoporosis age related w/current pathological fracture**

shoulder: unsp M80019- right M80011- left M80012-
humerus: unsp M80029- right M80021- left M80022-
forearm: unsp M80039- right M80031- left M80032-
hand: unsp M80049- right M80041- left M80042-
7th character indicates encounter/status
A - initial S - sequela D - subsequent routine healing
G - subsequent delayed healing
K - subsequent nonunion P - subsequent malunion

I770 **Arteriovenous fistula acquired**

T82390- **Arteriovenous shunt clot/malfunction/mechanical failure**

infected T827XX -
7th character indicates encounter
A- initial encounter D- subsequent encounter S- sequela

**Artery disorders**

septic embolism I76 arteriovenous fistula I770
narrowing / stricture I771 rupture / ulcer I772
fibromuscular dysplasia I773
necrosis I775 arteritis NOS I776
unspecified I779

I7779 **Artery dissection NOS other**

carotid I7771 iliac I7772
renal I7773 vertebral I7774

M2550 **Arthralgia NOS**

shoulder: right M25511 left M25512 unsp M25519
elbow: right M25521 left M25522 unsp M25529
wrist: right M25531 left M25532 unsp M25539
hip: right M25551 left M25552 unsp M25559
knee: right M25561 left M25562 unsp M25569
ankle & foot: right M25571 left M25572 unsp M25579

M129 **Arthritis NOS**

B779 **Ascariasis unspecified**

w/intestinal complications B770
w/pneumonia B7781
w/other complication B7789

R87611 **ASC-H: atypical squamous cells cannot exclude high grade squamous intrepithellal le**

R188 **Ascites abdominal / NOS / pseudochylous**

cardiac I509 chylous (nonfilarial) I898
d/t alcoholic: cirrhosis K7031 hepatits K7011
s. japonicum B652 malignant R180 in TB A1831

R87610 **ASC-US: atypical squamous cells of undetermined significance (from Pap smear)**

**I2510** **ASCVD: arteriosclerotic cardiovascular disease non hypertensive**

RELATED history of tobacco dependence Z87891

**Q211** **ASD: atrial septal defect acquired ostium secundum type II**

**I25810** **ASHD: arteriosclerotic heart disease of bypass graft NOS**

NOS w/unspecified angina pectoris I25799
transplanted heart NOS I25812
transplanted heart w/unspecified angina pectoris I25769
native coronary artery NOS I25110
native coronary artery w/unspecified angina pectoris I25119
native coronary artery with refractory angina I25112
unspecified coronary artery bypass w/refractory angina pectoris I25702
autologous vein coronary artery bypass w/refractory angina pectoris I25712
autologous coronary artery bypass w/refractory angina pectoris I25722
nonautologous biological coronary artery bypass graft(s) w/refractory angina pectoris I25
native coronary artery of transplanted heart with refractory angina pectoris I25752
bypass graft of coronary artery of transplanted heart w/refractory angina pectoris I25762
other coronary artery bypass graft(s) with refractory angina pectoris I25792
RELATED history of tobacco dependence Z87891

**E75249** **ASMD: Acid sphingomyelinase deficiency NOS**

ASMD type A E75240
ASMD type B E75241
ASMD type A/B E75244

**B449** **Aspergillosis unspecified**

Invasive pulmonary B440 Other pulmonary B441
Tonsillar B442 Disseminated / Generalized B447
Allergic bronchopulmonary B4481 Other B4489

**J8283** **Asthma eosinophilic**

Code first asthma by type

**J4520** **Asthma intermittent mild NOS**

w/acute exacerbation J4521 w/status asthmaticus J4522

**J4530** **Asthma persistent mild NOS**

w/acute exacerbation J4531 w/status asthmaticus J4532

**J4540** **Asthma persistent moderate NOS**

w/acute exacerbation J4541 w/status asthmaticus J4542

**J4550** **Asthma persistent severe NOS**

w/acute exacerbation J4551 w/status asthmaticus J4542

**Asthma unspecified & other**

unsp w/acute exacerbation J45901
unsp w/status asthmaticus J45902
unsp w/o complication J45909
exercise induced bronchospasm J45990
cough variant J45991 other J45998

R279 **Ataxia NOS**

cerebellar in other disease G3281
Friedreich's G1111 Early-onset unsp G1110
cerebral G3189 d/t CVA I69993
alcoholic G312 congenital nonprogressive G110
Ataxia-telangiectasia G118
Marie's/primary NOS/Sanger-Brown / late onset G112
w/defective DNA repair G113
locomotor progressive (neurosyphilis) A5211
Early-onset cerebellar ataxia with essential tremor / Hunt's ataxia G1119

N170 **ATN: acute tubular necrosis NOS**

I4820 **Atrial fibrillation chronic unspecified**

permanent I4821 NOS I4891
paroxysmal I480 persistent longstanding I4811
Persistent other I4819

I4892 **Atrial flutter NOS**

typical type I I483 atypical type II I484

I4430 **Atrioventricular block NOS**

1st degree I440 2nd degree I441
complete / 3rd degree I442 other I4439

E8582 **ATTR: transthyretin-related amyloidosis, Wild-type**

M049 **Autoinflammatory syndrome, unspecified**

Periodic fever syndromes M041
Cryopyrin-associated periodic syndromes M042
Other autoinflammatory syndromes M048

I4430 **AVB: atrioventricular block NOS**

complete I442

**Avitaminosis SEE Deficiency vitamin**

I471 **AVNRT: atrioventricular re-entrant nodal tachycardia**

also AVRT, AVT, PAT

R404 **Awareness altered transient**

L02411 **Axilla abscess cutaneous right, code organism if known**

left L02412

**L02431** **Axilla carbuncle right, code organism if known**

left L02432

**L02421** **Axilla furuncle/boil right, code organism if known**

left L02422

# B

**L02212** **Back abscess cutaneous, any part except buttock, code organism if known**

**L02232** **Back carbuncle, any part except buttock, code organism if known**

**L02222** **Back furuncle/boil, any part except buttock, code organism if known**

**M625A9** **Back muscle wasting and atrophy, not elsewhere classified unspecified level**

cervical M625A0 thoracic M625A1 lumbosacral M625A2

**L98429** **Back ulcer non-pressure chronic NOS**

limited to skin: L98421 fat layer exposed: L98422
muscle necrosis: L98423 bone necrosis: L98424
w/muscle involvement without necrosis L98425
w/bone involvement without necrosis L98426
with other specified severity L98425

**L8940** **Back ulcer pressure contiguous site of back, buttock & hip Unspecified**

Unstageable L8945 stage 1 L8941 stage 2 L8942
stage 3 L8943 stage 4 L8944
pressure-induced deep tissue damage L8946

**L89149** **Back ulcer pressure left lower NOS**

unstageable L89140 stage 1 L89141 stage 2 L89142
stage 3 L89143 stage 4 L89144
pressure induced deep tissue damage L89146

**L89129** **Back ulcer pressure left upper NOS**

unstageable L89120 stage 1 L89121 stage 2 L89122
stage 3 L89123 stage 4 L89124
pressure induced deep tissue damage L89126

**L89139** **Back ulcer pressure right lower NOS**

unstageable L89130 stage 1 L89131 stage 2 L89132
stage 3 L89133 stage 4 L89134
pressure induced deep tissue damage L89116

**L89109** **Back ulcer pressure unspecified area NOS**

unstageable L89100 stage 1 L89101 stage 2 L89102
stage 3 L89103 stage 4 L89104

**M549** **Backache NOS**

**R7881** **Bacteremia NOS code organism if known**

**R8271** **Bacteriuria**

**J45901** **BAIAE: bronchial asthma in acute exacerbation**

**Bladder catheter complication**

mechanical breakdown: cystostomy T83010- other T83018-
displacement: cystostomy T83020- other T83028-
leakage: cystostomy T83030- other T83038-
other mechanical: cystostomy T83090- other T83098-
infection/inflammation T8351X-
7th character indicates encounter
A- initial encounter D- subsequent encounter S- sequela

**Z466** **Bladder catheter fitting & adjustment**

**N312** **Bladder compliance high**

low compliance N318

**G9589** **Bladder cord NOS**

**N319** **Bladder disorder / dysfunction neurogenic / neuromuscular NOS**

**N329** **Bladder disorder NOS**

**N3289** **Bladder disorder other**

includes hemorrhage, hypertrophy, calcified, contracted

**N323** **Bladder diverticulum**

**R3914** **Bladder emptying incomplete if applicable/known code cause first**

**N808** **Bladder endometriosis**

**N80A0** **Bladder endometriosis NOS unspecified depth**

Superficial N80A1 Deep N80A2

**N3010** **Bladder fibrosis interstitial**

**R9341** **Bladder filling defect (found on imaging)**

**N322** **Bladder fistula NOS**

**D494** **Bladder growth NOS**

**N3289** **Bladder hemorrhage NOS**

**N3281** **Bladder hyperactivity/hypertonicity / overactive**

**N3289** **Bladder hyperemia**

**R32** **Bladder incontinence NOS**

functional / associated with cognitive impairment R3981
stress N393 urge N3941 overflow N39490
w/o sensory awareness N3942
nocturnal enuresis N3944 post-void dribbling N3943
continuous leakage N3945 mixed N3946
other / total / reflex N39498

**BLADDER INFECTION -- SEE CYSTITIS**

**N319** **Bladder instability**

**N318** **Bladder low compliance**

**N320** **Bladder neck contracture / obstruction / stenosis acquired**

RELATED bladder calculus N210

**C679** **Bladder neoplasm Malignant primary unsp / NOS**

trigone C670 dome C671 neck C675
lateral wall C672 anterior wall C673 urachus C677
posterior wall C674 ureteric orifice C676
overlapping sites C678
Secondary C7911 Benign D303
METS to bone C7951 mets to unsp lymph nodes C779

**N319** **Bladder neurogenic NOS**

d/t cauda equina syndrome G834
cord bladder NOS G9589

**Bladder neuropathic NEC**

uninhibited N310 reflex N311 flaccid N312

**N3281** **Bladder overactive**

**R3982** **Bladder pain chronic**

**N8110** **Bladder prolapse female NOS**

midline N8111 lateral N8112

**H01009** **Blepharitis NOS**

upper lid: right H01001 left H01004
lower lid: right H01002 left H01005
unsp lid: right HO1003 left H01006
upper & lower lids right H0100A left H0100B
Change 5th character if type known:
Ulcerative blepharitis = 1 Squamous blepharitis = 2

**G245** **Blepharospasm NOS**

d/t drugs G2401

**K902** **Blind Loop syndrome NOS**

postop K912

**R140** **Bloating**

**Blood Cell Count - SEE RBC or WBC**

**K921** **Blood in stool (melena)**

occult blood R195

**Blood pressure elevated diagnosis - SEE Hypertension**

**R030** **Blood pressure elevated w/o diagnosis of hypertension**

**R031** **Blood pressure reading low NOS**

**R6889** **Blood pressure unstable**

| | |
|---|---|
| | **Blood sugar SEE Glucose** |
| D892 | **BMH: benign monoclonal hypergammaglobulinemia** |
| | polyclonal (Waldenström) D890 |
| R948 | **BMR: basal metabolic rate abnormal** |
| N320 | **BNO: Bladder neck obstruction (acquired)** |
| | congenital Q6431<br>RELATED bladder calculus N210 |
| | **Boil - SEE furuncle at site** |
| M8560 | **Bone cyst degenerative/NOS unsp site** |
| | aneurysmal/solitary/unicameral unsp site M8540 |
| C7952 | **Bone marrow Mets/ secondary neoplasm** |
| M8700 | **Bone necrosis aseptic/avascular NOS unsp bone** |
| | SEE osteonecrosis at arm or leg |
| C7951 | **Bone neoplasm SECONDARY / Mets to bone** |
| | Mets to bone marrow C7952 |
| M779 | **Bone spur NOS** |
| | Calcaneal spur foot unsp M7730 right M7731 left M7732<br>Iliac crest spur unsp hip M7620 right M7621 left M7622<br>vertebrae spur M2578 |
| J8489 | **BOOP: bronchiolitis obliterans organizing pneumonia** |
| A051 | **Botulism NOS** |
| | **BOWEL -- ALSO see colon** |
| R194 | **Bowel habit change NOS** |
| K5641 | **Bowel impaction fecal** |
| | other K5649 |
| K589 | **Bowel irritable NOS (IBS)** |
| | w/diarrhea K580 constipation K581 mixed K582 other K588 |
| K592 | **Bowel neurogenic NOS** |
| K56609 | **Bowel obstruction NOS** |
| | Partial unspecified as to cause K56600<br>Complete unspecified as to cause K56601<br>Other partial intestinal obstruction K56690<br>Other complete intestinal obstruction K56691<br>Other unspecified as to partial vs complete K56699<br>Postop unspecified as to partial vs complete K9130<br>Postop partial K9131 Postop complete K9132 |
| K560 | **Bowel paralytic ileus** |

**Bowel sounds**

absent R1911 hyperactive R1912 abnormal NOS R1915

K562 **Bowel volvulus includes strangulation, torsion, twist**

N400 **BPH: benign prostatic hypertrophy NOS**

with lower urinary tract symptoms (LUTS) N401
Also code applicable LUTS below
bladder incomplete emptying R3914 frequency R350
nocturia physical R351 psychogenic F458
straining on urination R3916 hesitancy R3911
urinary obstruction N139 retention R339
urgency N3941 weak urinary stream R3912
urinary incontinence NOS R32 see urinary incontinence for more

H8110 **BPPV: benign positional paroxysmal vertigo NOS unsp**

bilat H8113 right ear H8111 left ear H8112

Z4689 **Brace orthopedic fitting & adjustment**

R001 **Bradycardia NOS**

G060 **Brain abscess and/or granuloma NOS**

in TB A1781 amebic A066
chromomycotic B431 gonococcal A5482

N611 **Breast abscess acute/chronic/nonpuerperal Includes Mastitis w/abscess**

N6089 **Breast cyst sebaceous NOS**

solitary N6009 cystic/fibrocystic N6019
Change final character if breast is known: right =1 left = 2

N6029 **Breast fibroadenosis unspecified**

right N6021 left N6022

N6019 **Breast fibrocystic unspecified**

right N6011 left N6012

N6039 **Breast fibrosclerosis unspecified**

right N6031 left N6032

N630 **Breast lesion/lump/mass NOS**

**Breast lump/mass unspecified severity, specified location**

unspec quad right N6310 left N6320
upper outer quad right N6311 left N6321
upper inner quad right N6312 left N6322
lower outer quad right N6313 left N6323
lower inner quad right N6314 left N6324
Overlapping quads right N6315 left N6325
axillary tail right N6331 left N6332
subareolar right N6341 left N6342

**Breast neoplasm MALIGNANT Primary female (code for male = change 5th charact**

nipple & areola: unsp C50019 right C50011 left C50012
central portion: unsp C50119 right C50111 left C50112
upper inner quad: unsp C50219 right C50211 left C50212
lower inner quad: unsp C50319 right C50311 left C50312
upper outer quad: unsp C50419 right C50411 left C50412
lower outer quad: unsp C50519 right C50511 left C50512
axillary tail: unsp C50619 right C50611 left C50612
overlapping sites: unsp C50819 right C50811 left C50812
unspecified site: unsp C50919 right C50911 left C50912

**Breast neoplasm Secondary and benign (female or male)**

Secondary any site C7981
benign: unsp D249 right D241 left D242
Mets to axilla / arm lymph node C773

**N644** **Breast pain NOS**

**Z4430** **Breast prosthesis fitting & adjustment NOS**

right Z4431 left Z4432

**Broad ligament disorders**

cyst N838 endometriosis N803 hematoma N837
disorder noninflammatory N839 laceration syndrome N838

**Broad ligament neoplasm**

MALIGNANT primary unsp C5710 right C5711 left C5712
Secondary C7982 Benign D282
Mets to bone C7951 METS to unsp lymph nodes C779
Mets to intraabdominal lymph node C772
Mets to intrapelvic lymph node C775

**J479** **Bronchiectasis NOS**

w/acute lower resp infection J470
w/acute exacerbation J471
Code also to identify infection, if applicable

**J219** **Bronchiolitis ACUTE unspecified**

d/t respiratory synctial virus J210
d/t human metapneumovirus J211
d/t other specified organism J218

**J209** **Bronchitis acute NOS**

Mycoplasma pneumoniae J200 Hemophilus influenzae J201
streptococcus J202 coxsackie virus J203
parainfluenza virus J204 respiratory syncytial virus J205
rhinovirus J206 echovirus J207
other specified organisms J208

**J42** **Bronchitis chronic NOS**

chronic simple J410 chronic mucopurulent J411
chronic mixed simple mucopurulent J418

**J40** **Bronchitis NOS**

RELATED
hx of tobacco use Z87891 tobacco use Z720
exp to environmental smoke NOS Z7722
exp to environmental smoke occupational Z5731

**J984** **Broncholithiasis**

**J9801** **Bronchospasm acute NOS**

exercise induced J45990
w/bronchitis code bronchitis
w/acute bronchiolitis code bronchiolitis

**G8381** **Brown-Sequard syndrome**

**A239** **Brucellosis NOS**

d/t Brucella melitensis A230 d/t Brucella abortus A231
d/t Brucella suis A232 d/t Brucella canis A233
Other A238

**I498** **Brugada syndrome**

**I820** **Budd-Chiari syndrome**

**F502** **Bulemia nervosa / NOS**

**I454** **Bundle branch block NOS -- SEE heart block for more**

trifascicular I453 -- SEE heart block for more

**M21619** **Bunion unspecified foot**

right M21611 left M21612

**M21629** **Bunionette unspecified foot**

right M21621 left M21622

**C8370** **Burkitt lymphoma unspecified site**

lymph nodes of head, face, and neck C8371
intrathoracic lymph nodes C8372
intra-abdominal lymph nodes C8373
lymph nodes of axilla and arm C8374
lymph nodes of inguinal region and leg C8375
intrapelvic lymph nodes C8376
spleen C8377 lymph nodes of multiple sites C8378
extranodal and solid organ sites C8379

**M719** **Bursitis NOS**

**L0231** **Buttock abscess cutaneous**

**L0233** **Buttock carbuncle**

**L0232** **Buttock furuncle/boil**

**L98419** **Buttock ulcer non-pressure chronic NOS**

limited to skin L98411 w/fat layer exposed L98412
w/muscle necrosis L98413 w/bone necrosis L98414
w/ muscle involvement without necrosis L98415
w/ bone involvement without necrosis L98416
w/ other specified severity L98418

**Buttock ulcer pressure contiguous site of back, buttock & hip SEE BACK ulcer press**

**L89329** **Buttock ulcer pressure left NOS**

unstageable L89320
stage 1 L89321 stage 2 L89322
stage 3 L89323 stage 4 L89324
pressure-induced deep tissue damage L89326

**L89319** **Buttock ulcer pressure right NOS**

unstageable L89310
stage 1 L89311 stage 2 L89312
stage 3 L89313 stage 4 L89314
pressure-induced deep tissue damage L89316

**L89309** **Buttock ulcer pressure unspecified side NOS**

unstageable L89300
stage 1 L89301 stage 2 L89302
stage 3 L89303 stage 4 L89304
pressure-induced deep tissue damage L89306

# C

**Z951** **CABG status**

**R64** **Cachexia NOS Code underlying condition first if known**

of old age R54

**I2510** **CAD: coronary artery disease NOS**

RELATED history of tobacco dependence Z87891

**I67850** **CADASIL (Cerebral autosomal dominant arteriopathy with subcortical infarcts &**

**E8350** **Calcium metabolism disorder NOS**

hypocalcemia E8351 hypercalcemia E8352 other E8359

**L97229** **Calf ulcer non-pressure chronic LEFT NOS**

limited to skin L97221 w/fat layer exposed L97222
w/muscle necrosis L97223 w/bone necrosis L97224
w/muscle involvement w/o necrosis L97225
w/bone involvement w/o necrosis L97226
w/other specified severity L97228
RIGHT - change 5th digit to1
UNSPECIFIED SIDE - change 5th digit to 0

**B379** **Candidiasis NOS**

esophagus B3781 lung B371 vagina/vulva B373
disseminated/systemic/sepsis B377
skin/nails B372 stomatitis/oral B370
ear/ otitis B3784 proctitis B3782 other/osteomyelitis B3789
meningitis B375 endocarditis B376 cheilitis B3783

**K120** **Canker sore**

**T40714-** **Cannabis Poisoning undetermined nature**

accidental (unintentional) T40711-
intentional self-harm T40712-
assault T40713-
adverse effect T40715-
underdosing T40716-
FOR synthetic cannabinoids CHANGE 5TH character to 2
Add7th character for encounter
A - initial encounter D - subsequent encounter S - sequela

**H9325** **CAPD: central auditory processing disorder**

**M779** **Capsulitis NOS**

**I499** **Cardiac arrythmia / dysrhythmia NOS**

**T827XX -** **Cardiac device internal infected NOS**

infected cardiac valve prosthesis T826xx -
7th character indicates encounter
A - initial encounter D - subsequent encounter S - sequela

**I517** **Cardiac dilatation / hypertrophy NOS**

| | |
|---|---|
| **I509** | **Cardiac failure NOS** |
| **R012** | **Cardiac friction fremitus / precordial friction / dullness** |
| **I97111** | **Cardiac insufficiency postop NOS** |
| | following cardiac surgery I97110 |
| **I249** | **Cardiac ischemia acute NOS** |
| **R011** | **Cardiac murmur NOS** |
| | Benign and innocent murmurs R010<br>Other cardiac sounds R012 |
| **Z950** | **Cardiac pacemaker dependence** |
| **I510** | **Cardiac septal defect acquired as sequelae to myocardial infarction old** |
| **I517** | **Cardiomegaly** |
| **I429** | **Cardiomyopathy NOS** |
| | Congestive I420 obstructive hypertrophic I421 other hyertrophic I422<br>endomyocardial/eosinophilic I423 constrictive NOS I425<br>congenital I424 alcoholic I426 other I428<br>d/t drug/external agent I427 stress induced I5181<br>Gout cardiomyopathy I43<br>ischemic I255 May USE WITH i42 codes |
| **I5189** | **Carditis NOS** |
| | rheumatic: acute I019 NOS I099<br>coxsackie virus NOS B3320 meningococcal NOS A3950 |
| **B3320** | **CarditisViral (Coxsackie virus) unspecified** |
| | endocarditis B3321 myocarditis B3322<br>pericarditis B3323 cardiomyopathy B3324 |
| **Z515** | **Care palliative** |
| **Z742** | **Caregiver not available** |
| **I720** | **Carotid artery aneurysm** |
| **I7771** | **Carotid artery dissection** |
| **G451** | **Carotid artery insufficiency** |
| **I6529** | **Carotid artery occlusion / stenosis NOS** |
| | right I6521 left I6522 bilat I6423 |
| **G9001** | **Carotid sinus syncope / syndrome** |
| **G5600** | **Carpal tunnel syndrome NOS** |
| | right arm G5601 left arm G5602 bilateral G5603 |
| | **Cast ulcer SEE pressure ulcer at site** |

**D47Z2** **Castleman disease**

If applicable code also hhv B infection B1089
If appllcable may also code Kaposi's sarcoma
See Kaposi for a list of site codes
if applicable,code human herpesvirus 8 infection B1089

**Cataract age related**

morgagnian unsp H2520 bilat H2523 right H2521 left H2522
nuclear unsp H2510 bilat H2513 right H2511 left H2512
combined types unsp H25819 bilat H25813 right H25811 left H25812
cortical unsp H25019 bilat H25013 right H25011 left H25012
anterior subcapsular unsp H25039 bilat H25033 right H25031 left H25032

**H269** **Cataract NOS**

drug induced unsp H2630 bilat H2633 right H2631 left H2632
unspec traumatic unsp H26109 bilat H26103 right H26101 left H26102

**F061** **Catatonia NOS Includes d/t known physiological condition or associated with another**

Code underlying condition first
If applicable also code catatonic schizophrenia F202

**T80219 -** **Catheter central venous, infection unspecified type**

systemic infection T80211- local infection T80212-
other specified T80218 -
7th character indicates encounter
A - initial encounter D - subsequent encounter S - sequela
includes Hickman, PIC, portacath, triple lumen, pulmonary artery catheter

**Catheter fitting & adjustment**

vascular Z452 nonvascular Z4682
extracorporeal dialysis Z4901 peritoneal dialysis Z4902

**G834** **Cauda equina syndrome**

**Causalgia SEE arm or leg**

**F09** **CBS: chronic brain syndrome**

**N3020** **CC: chronic cystitis NOS**

w/hematuria N3021 chronic interstitial NOS N3010
chronic interstitial w/hematuria N3011

**N80539** **Cecum endometriosis NOS unspecified depth**

Superficial N80531 Deep N80532

**I774** **Celiac artery compression syndrome**

**K900** **Celiac disease**

Code also exocrine pancreatic insufficiency K8681

**R82998** **Cells and casts in urine**

**I671** **Cerebral aneurysm NOS nonruptured**

**I670** **Cerebral artery dissection nonruptured**

**I6619** **Cerebral artery occlusion & stenosis w/o infarction Anterior NOS**
right I6611 left I6612 bilat I6613

**I6609** **Cerebral artery occlusion & stenosis w/o infarction Middle NOS**
right I6601 left I6602 bilat I6603

**I669** **Cerebral artery occlusion & stenosis w/o infarction NOS**
other I668

**I6629** **Cerebral artery occlusion & stenosis w/o infarction Posterior NOS**
right I6621 left I6622 bilat I6623

**G460** **Cerebral artery syndrome middle**
anterior G461 posterior G462

**I672** **Cerebral atherosclerosis**

**G936** **Cerebral edema**

**I619** **Cerebral hemorrhage unspecified**

**I6340** **Cerebral infarction d/t cerebral artery EMBOLISM NOS**
middle: right I63411 left I63412 NOS I63419
anterior: right I63421 left I63422 NOS I63429
posterior: right I63431 left I63432 NOS I63439
cerebellar: right I63441 left I63442 NOS I63449
If known code NIH stroke score

**I6350** **Cerebral infarction d/t cerebral artery OCCLUSION/STENOSIS NOS**
middle: right I63511 left I63512 NOS I63519
anterior: right I63521 left I63522 NOS I63529
posterior: right I63531 left I63532 NOS I63539
cerebellar: right I63541 left I63542 NOS I63549
If known code NIH stroke score

**I6330** **Cerebral infarction d/t cerebral artery THROMBOSIS NOS**
middle: right I63511 left I63512 NOS I63519
anterior: right I63521 left I63522 NOS I63529
posterior: right I63531 left I63532 NOS I63539
cerebellar: right I63541 left I63542 NOS I63549
If known code NIH stroke score

**I6330** **Cerebral infarction d/t cerebral artery THROMBOSIS NOS**
middle: right I63311 left I63312 NOS I63319
anterior: right I63321 left I63322 NOS I63329
posterior: right I63331 left I63332 NOS I63339
cerebellar: right I63341 left I63342 NOS I63349
If known code NIH stroke score

**I6310** **Cerebral infarction d/t precerebral artery EMBOLISM NOS**

vertebral artery: right I63111 left I63112 NOS I63119
carotid artery: right I63131 left I63132 NOS I63139
basilar artery I6312 other I6319
If known code NIH stroke score

**I6320** **Cerebral infarction d/t precerebral artery OCCLUSION/STENOSIS NOS**

vertebral artery: right I63211 left I63.212 NOS I63219
carotid artery: right I63231 left I63232 NOS I63239
basilar artery I6322 other I6329
If known code NIH stroke score

**I6300** **Cerebral infarction d/t precerebral artery THROMBOSIS NOS**

vertebral artery: right I63011 left I63012 NOS I63019
carotid artery: right I63031 left I63032 NOS I63039
basilar artery I6302 other I6309
If known code NIH stroke score

**I69359** **Cerebral infarction late effect hemiplegia NOS**

dominant side: right I69351 left I69352
nondominant side: right I59353 left I69354

**Cerebral Infarction RELATED stroke score, National Institutes of Health Stroke Scal**

Code first the type of cerebral infarction (I63-)
R29700 NIHSS score 0 R29701 NIHSS score 1
R29702 NIHSS score 2 R29703 NIHSS score 3
Scores range from 0 to 42 using pattern above
R297xx where xx equals the score

**I6930** **Cerebral infarction sequelae NOS (sequelae to stroke NOS)**

aphasia I69320 dysphasia I69321
dysarthria I69322 fluency disorder I69323
apraxia I69390 dysphagia I69391
facial weakness/droop I69392 ataxia I69393
cognitive deficits I6931
RELATED history of tobacco dependence Z87891

**I6782** **Cerebral ischemia**

**G809** **Cerebral palsy NOS**

spastic: quadriplegic G800 diplegic G801 hemiplegic G802
athetoid G803 ataxic G804 other G808

**G9600** **Cerebrospinal fluid leak unspecified**

Cranial cerebrospinal fluid leak, spontaneous G9601
Spinal cerebrospinal fluid leak, spontaneous G9602
Other cranial cerebrospinal fluid leak G9608
Other spinal cerebrospinal fluid leak G9609
SEE spinal puncture for leak as complication

**I639** **Cerebrovascular accident acute/NOS (stroke)**

d/t cerebral venous thrombosis nonpyogenic I636
d/t occlusion NOS I6359 other NEC I638

**Cerebrovascular disease late effect monoplegia**

unspecified side: arm I69339 leg I69349
dominant arm: right I69331 left I69332
nondominant arm: right I69333 left I69334
dominant leg: right I69341 left I69342
nondominant leg: right I69343 left I69344

**I6990** **Cerebrovascular disease late effect NOS**

aphasia I69920 apraxia I69990
ataxia I69993 facial weakness I69992
dysphagia I69991 dysphasia I69923
fluency/ vertigo /sensation / vision / other I69998
for I69998 use additional code to SPECIFY which
RELATED history of tobacco dependence Z87891

**I69919** **Cerebrovascular disease unspecified late effects cognitive deficits**

Attention and concentration deficit I69910
Memory deficit I69911 Psychomotor deficit I69913
Visuospatial deficit and spatial neglect I698912
Frontal lobe and executive function deficit I69914
Cognitive social or emotional deficit I69915
Other symptoms and signs involving cognitive functions I69918
Speech and language, fluency disorder I69923

**I69319** **Cerebrovascular disease unspecified late effects cognitive deficits**

Attention and concentration deficit I69910
Memory deficit I69911 Psychomotor deficit I69913
Visuospatial deficit and spatial neglect I698912
Frontal lobe and executive function deficit I69914
Cognitive social or emotional deficit I69915
Other symptoms and signs involving cognitive functions I69918
Speech and language, fluency disorder I69923

**I679** **Cerebrovascular disease, unspecified**

**I679** **Cerebrovascular disease, unspecified**

**I6781** **Cerebrovascular insufficiency acute**

**I6781** **Cerebrovascular insufficiency acute**

**I69319** **Cerebrral infarction Late effects sequelae cognitive deficits Unspecified symptoms an**

Attention and concentration deficit I69310
Memory deficit I69311
Visuospatial deficit and spatial neglect I69312
Psychomotor deficit I69313
Frontal lobe and executive function deficit I69314
Cognitive social or emotional deficit I69315
Other symptoms and signs involving cognitive functions I69318
Speech and language, fluency disorder I69323

**H6120** **Cerumen impacted unspecified**

right H6121 left H6122 bilat H6123

**M5382** **Cervical syndrome acute (spine)**

**M542** **Cervicalgia NOS**

**N72** **Cervicitis NOS**

Gonococcal A5403 Chlamydial A5609

**Z90710** **Cervix absence w/absence of uterus acquired**

w/ remaining uterus Z90712

**N881** **Cervix adhesions/bands incl cicatrix (old postpartum)**

**N888** **Cervix disorder noninflammatory other also atrophy/cyst/fibrosis**

unspecified noninflammatory cervix disorder N889

**N879** **Cervix dysplasia NOS**

mild (CIN type I) N870
moderate (CIN type II) N871
CIN type III D069

**N86** **Cervix ectropion/erosion/eversion aka trophic ulcer**

**N884** **Cervix elongation hypertrophic**

**N8000** **Cervix endometriosis unspecified**

Superficial N8001 Deep N8002
Adenomyosis N8003

**N888** **Cervix fibrosis**

**N883** **Cervix incompetence**

**Cervix neoplasm**

MALIGNANT primary: endocervix C530 exocervix C531
MALIGNANT primary: overlapping sites C538 unspecified/NOS C539
Secondary C7982 Benign C260
Mets to bone C7951 Mets to intraabdominal lymph node C772
mets to unspecified lymph nodes C779
Mets to intrapelvic lymph node C775

**N841** **Cervix polyp mucous / NOS**

**N882** **Cervix stenosis/stricture**

**N812** **Cervix stump prolapse**

**E849** **CF: cystic fibrosis NOS**

pulmonary E840 intestinal except meconium E8419
meconium ileus E8411 other E848
Code Also exocrine pancreatic insufficiency K8681

**G9332** **CFS: chronic fatigue syndrome**

postviral fatigue syndrome G9331
Other post infection and related fatigue syndromes G9339

**G44009** **CHA: cluster headache NOS (also just CH)**

**B571** **Chagas' disease acute NOS**

acute w/heart involvement B570
chronic w/heart involvement B572
w/digestive system involvement unspecified B5730
w/megaesophagus B5731 w/megacolon B5732
w/other digestive system involvement B5739
w/nervous system involvement, unspecified B5740
w/meningitis B5741 w/meningoencephalitis B5742
w/other nervous system involvement B5749
w/ organ involvement other B575

**G600** **Charcot-Marie-Tooth disease**

**Q249** **CHD: congenital heart disease NOS**

**Z5111** **Chemotherapy antineoplastic as reason for visit**

**T8149x -** **Chest tube site infection NOS**

7th character indicates encounter
A - initial encounter D - subsequent encounter S - sequela

**I509** **CHF: congestive heart failure NOS SEE Heart failure congestive for more**

**A980** **CHF: Congo/Crimean hemorrhagic fever (Congo virus)**

**S069X9-** **CHI: closed head injury unspecified nature NOS**

no LOC S069X0- LOC =< 30 min S069X1-
LOC 31-59 min S069X2- LOC 1-5 hrs S069X3-
LOC = loss of consciousness
7th character indicates encounter
A - initial encounter D - subsequent encounter S - sequela
If dementia present code also one:
without behavioral disturbance F0280
with behavioral disturbance F0281

**B019** **Chickenpox NOS**

w/complication other B0189 w/keratitis B0181
w/encephalitis B0111 w/meningitis B010
w/pneumonia B012 w/myelitis B0112

**R6883** **Chills NOS**

w/fever R509

**A749** **Chlamydial infection unspecified**

genitourinary tract unspecified A562
of lower genitourinary tract unspecified A5600
For other SEE condition/diagnosis

**K8309** **Cholangitis acute/ascending/chronic/NOS/recurrent/suppurative**

chronic nonsuppurative destructive K743
primary sclerosing cholangitis K8301

**K819** **Cholecystitis NOS**

acute K810 chronic K811 acute w/chronic K812

**K8020** **Cholelithiasis NOS**

obstructed K8021

**K8000** **Cholelithiasis w/acute cholecystitis NOS**

obstructed K8001
w/chronic cholecystis: NOS K8010 obstructed K8011
w/chronic & acute cholecystitis: NOS K8012 obstructed K8013
w/other cholecystitis: NOS K8018 obstructed K8019
RELATED Gangrene K82A1 Perforation K82A2

**A009** **Cholera NOS**

d/t Vibrio cholerae 01, biovar cholerae A000
d/t Vibrio cholerae 01, biovar eltor A001

**H61039** **Chondritis ear external NOS**

right H61031 left H61032 bilat H61033

**G255** **Chorea other / NOS**

drug induced G254

**G9332** **Chronic fatigue syndrome chronic NOS**

**M301** **Churg-Strauss**

**I3131** **Chylopericardium Malignant pericardial effusion in diseases classified elsewhere**

Other pericardial effusion (noninflammatory) I3139

**I898** **Chylous ascites / cyst**

**G6181** **CIDP: chronic inflammatory demyelinating polyneuropathy**

**N879** **CIN: cervix interstitial neoplasia NOS histologically confirmed**

type I mild N870 type II moderate N871 type III D069

**K0530** **CIPD: chronic inflammatory periodontal disease NOS**

localized K0531 generalized K0532

**A8100** **CJD: Creutzfeldt-Jakob disease NOS**

familial, iatrogenic specified NEC A8109
variant A8101 (CJDv or v CJD)

**N189** **CKD: chronic kidney disease NOS**

stage I N181 stage II (mild) N182
stage III (moderate) unspecified N1830
stage III (moderate) stage 3a N1831
stage III (moderate) stage 3b N1832
stage IV (severe) N184 stage V N185
stage V requiring chronic dialysis (ESRD) N186
RELATED Anemia in chronic kidney disease D631

**I739** **Claudication intermittent NOS**

w/atherosclerosis of the extremities NOS I70219
w/atherosclerosis of leg: right I70211 left I70212 bilat I70213

**R294** **Clicking hip**

**C9110** **CLL: chronic lymphoid leukemia NOS**

in remission C9111 in relapse C9112

**A047-** **Clostridium difficile entercolitis**

Requires 5th character 1=recurrent 2=not specified as recurrent

**G600** **CMT: Charcot-Marie-Tooth disease**

**B259** **CMV: cytomegalic virus local/systemic infection NOS**

pneumonitis B250 hepatitis B251
pancreatitis B252 other B258
mononucleosis NOS B2710
mono w/polyneuropathy B2711 mono w/meningitis B271
mono w/ other complication NEC B2719

**R791** **Coagulation profile abnormal (Low von Willebrand factor)**

**S322xx -** **Coccyx fracture Other (and transverse)**

Add the appropriate 7th character:
initial encounter: closed fracture = A open fracture = B
subsequent encounter: routine healing = D delayed healing = G
subsequent encounter fracture w/ nonunion = K
sequela = S

**J678** **Coffee worker's lung**

**R419** **Cognitive function altered NOS**

attention / concentration deficit R41840
communicative deficit R41841
visuospatial deficit R41842
psychomotor deficit R41843
executive function/frontal lobe deficit R41844
altered mental status NOS R4182
age-related decline R4181
Cognitive impairment mild, so stated G3184
Do not use these with codes for sequelae of cerebral hemmorhage

**J00** **Cold common aka acute rhinitis, coryza, acute nasopharyngitis**

**J449** **COLD: chronic obstructive lung/pulmonary disease NOS (COPD)**

ncludes w/asthma, bronchitis NOS, and emphysema
w/acute lower respiratory infection J440
w/acute exacerbation J441
Also code infection and asthma if presen

**R1084** **Colic NOS adult**

**A09** **Colitis infectious/septic/ presumed infectious NOS**

C. dificile / pseudomembranous A047
protozoal NOS A079 amebic nondysenteric A062

**K559** **Colitis ischemic NOS**

acute K550 chronic K55

**K5150** **Colitis left sided NOS**

w/rectal bleeding K51511
w/intestinal obstruction K51512
w/fistula K51513 w/abscess K51514
other specified complicaton K51518
w/unspecified complication K51519

**K529** **Colitis noninfective NOS**

granulomatous/regional/transmural K5010 (Crohn's)
d/t radiation K520 eosinophilic K5282
adaptive/membranous/mucous K589
allergic / dietetic K522 drug induced / toxic K521

**K5190** **Colitis ulcerative NOS**

w/rectal bleeding K51911
w/intestinal obstruction K51912
w/fistula K51913 w/abscess K51914
w/other specified complication K51918
w/unsp complication K51919
RELATED arthritis or polyarthritis M0200

**M359** **Collagen disease NOS/non vascular**

vascular M310

| | |
|---|---|
| **S52539-** | **Colles' fracture (radius) unspecified** |
| | right S52531- left S52532-<br>7th character indicates encounter/status<br>A - initial S - sequela<br>D - subsequent routine healing K - subsequent nonunion<br>G - subsequent delayed healing P - subsequent malunion |
| **K630** | **Colon abscess** |
| **K660** | **Colon adhesions** |
| **K5989** | **Colon atonic/atony** |
| **K5939** | **Colon dilatation** |
| | **Colon diverticular disease** |
| | diverticulitis w/perforation & abscess K5720<br>diverticulitis w/perforation & abscess w/bleeding K5721<br>diverticulitis: NOS K5732 w/bleeding K5733<br>diverticulosis: NOS K5730 w/bleeding K5731 |
| **K5010** | **Colon enteritis regional NOS** |
| | SEE Crohn's disease large intestine for more<br>Regional enteritis NOS K5090 |
| **K632** | **Colon fistula NOS** |
| **K560** | **Colon ileus paralytic** |
| **K5641** | **Colon impaction fecal** |
| | other K5649 |
| **K55049** | **Colon infarction Acute extent unspecified (Gangrene, Necrosis)** |
| | Focal K55041 Diffuse K55042 |
| **K561** | **Colon intussusception/invagination** |
| **K589** | **Colon irritable** |
| | w/diarrhea K580 w/ constipation K581<br>Mixed K582 Other K588 |
| **K55039** | **Colon ischemia Acute (reversible) extent unspecified** |
| | Focal K55031 Diffuse K55032 |

**Colon neoplasm**

MALIGNANT primary
cecum C180 appendix C181
ascending colon C182 hepatic flexure C183
descending colon C186 sigmoid colon C187
overlapping sites C188 unspecified C189
SECONDARY C785
BENIGN
cecum D120 appendix D121 ascending colon D122
transverse colon D123 descending colon D124
sigmoid colon D125 unspecified/NOS D126

**K592** **Colon neurogenic**

**N80559** **Colon NOS endometriosis NOS unspecified depth**

Superficial N80551 Deep N80552

**K56609** **Colon obstruction/occlusion/stenosis/stricture NOS unspecified partial or complete**

Partial unspecified as to cause K56600
Complete unspecified as to cause K56601
Other partial intestinal obstruction K56690
Other complete intestinal obstruction K56691
Other unspecified as to partial vs complete K56699
Postop unspecified as to partial vs complete K9130
Postop partial K9131 Postop complete K9132

**K560** **Colon paralysis**

**K631** **Colon perforation nontraumatic**

**Z86010** **Colon polyp history**

**K635** **Colon polyp NOS**

Adenomatous polyp / polyposis D126
Inflammatory NOS K5140
Inflammatory w/ rectal bleeding K51411
Inflammatory w/ intestinal obstruction K51412
Inflammatory w/ fistula K51413
Inflammatory w/ abscess K51414
Inflammatory w/ other complication K51418
Inflammatory w/ unspecified complications K51419

**K589** **Colon spastic**

w/diarrhea K580 w/constipation K581
Mixed K582 Other K588

**K562** **Colon volvulus - includes strangulation, torsion, twist**

**Z433** **Colostomy care, closure/takedown, toilet/cleansing**

status w/o need for care Z933
fitting & adjust Z4659

**K9400** **Colostomy complication NOS**

hemorrhage K9401 malfunction K9403
other K9409 infection K9402
for infection also code type eg. abd wall cellulitis L03311 or a sepsis
granulation of surrounding skin L928

**Compartment syndrome nontraumatic**

unspecified or other M79A9 abdomen M79A3
Leg: unsp M79A29 right M79A21 left M79A22
Arm: unsp M79A19 right M79A11 left M79A12

**COMPLEX REGIONAL Pain Syndrome -SEE CRPS above**

**Compression fracture SEE site**

**Z7401** **Confined to bed**

**R410** **Confusion NOS**

Confusion organic acute/subacute/NOS F05

**I509** **Congestive heart failure NOS - SEE heart failure congestive for more**

**A740** **Conjunctivitis Chlamydial**

**H10829** **Conjunctivitis rosacea unspecified**

right eye H10821 left eye H10822 bilateral H10823
Code first underlying rosacea dermatitis
Rosacea -- unspecified L719 Other rosacea L718
Rhinophyma L711 Perioral dermatitis L710

**H10239** **Conjunctivitis serous except viral NOS**

right eye H10231 left eye H10232 bilateral H10233

**H1030** **Conjunctivitis unspecified acute unspecified eye**

right eye H1031 left eye H1032 bilateral H1033

**H10409** **Conjunctivitis unspecified chronic, unspecified eye**

right eye H10401 left eye H10402 bilateral H10403

**B309** **Conjunctivitis viral NOS**

keratoconjunctivitis d/t adenovirus B300
conjunctivitis d/t adenovirus B301
pharyngoconjunctivitis B302
acute epidemic hemorrhagic conjunctivitis B303
other viral / Newcastle B308

**K5900** **Constipation NOS**

slow transit K5901 outlet dysfunction K5902
other K5909 fecal impaction K5641
incomplete defecation R150
psychogenic F458 Drug induced K5903
Chronic idiopathic / Functional K5904

**M2450** **Contractures NOS SEE site if known**

**Z5189** **Convalescence following radiotherapy**

**R569** **Convulsions NOS**

febrile NOS R5600 febrile complex R5601
post traumatic R561

**R279** **Coordination lack of NOS**

ataxia NOS R270 other R278

**I2609** **Cor pulmonale acute NOS**

chronic NOS I2781
acute w/saddle embolus of pulmonary artery I2602
acute w/septic pulmonary embolism I2601

**G9589** **Cord bladder NOS**

**E7403** **Cori disease**

**I2510** **Coronary artery atherosclerosis native artery NOS**

w/unstable angina I25110 w/refractory angina I25112
w/angina & documented spasm I25111
w/other angina I25118 w/unspecified angina I25119
RELATED
atherosclerosis d/t lipid rich plaque I2583
atherosclerosis d/t calcified coronary lesion I2584
history of tobacco dependence Z87891

**Z951** **Coronary artery bypass graft status**

**I2542** **Coronary artery dissection**

**Coronary artery occlusion**

chronic total occlusion I2582
acute not resulting in MI I240

**B342** **Coronavirus infection unspecified**

DO NOT USE WITH pneumonia due to SARS-associated coronavirus
COVID-19 U071 do not use with other corona virus codes
SARS-associated coronavirus as the cause of diseases classified elsewhere B9721
Other coronavirus as the cause of diseases classified elsewhere B9729
Pneumonia due to SARS-associated coronavirus J1281

**R059** **Cough NOS**

psychogenic F458 smoker's J410 w/hemorrhage NOS R042
Acute R051 Subacute R052
Chronic/Persistent/Unexplained R053
Cough syncope R054 Code first syncope and collapse (R55)
Other specified R058

**Z7182** **Counseling exercise**

**U071** **COVID-19**

**U099** **COVID-19 post infection condition**

RELATED Code first if known
loss of smell / taste R438
multisystem inflammatory syndrome M3581
pulmonary fibrosis J8410
Pulmonary embolism NOS I2699
Septic pulmonary embolism w/o acute cor pulmonale I2690
saddle embolus of pulmonary artery w/o acute cor pulmonale I2692
Single subsegmental pulmonary embolism w/o acute cor pulmonale I2693
Multiple subsegmental pulmonary emboli w/o acute cor pulmonale I2694
Chronic respiratory failure, unspecified J9610
Chronic respiratory failure with hypoxia J9611
Chronic respiratory failure with hypercapnia J9612

**N340** **Cowper's gland abscess**

**B3320** **Coxsackie virus carditis unspecified**

endocarditis B3321 myocarditis B3322
pericarditis B3323 cardiomyopathy B3324

**G809** **CP: cerebral palsy NOS**

mixed / other G808 athetoid G803 ataxic G804
spastic: quadriplegic G800 diplegic / NOS G801 hemiplegic G80

**M96A9** **CPR Injury other ffracture associated with CPR**

sternum M96A1
one rib M96A2
Multiple fractures of ribs M96A3
Flail chest M96A4

**G890** **CPS: central pain syndrome**

**R252** **Cramp in limbs NOS**

Charley-horse M6283
muscle spasm of back M62830
carpopedal spasm R290
cramps leg sleep related G4762

**T672XX -** **Cramps heat**

7th character indicates encounter
A - initial encounter D - subsequent encounter S - sequela

**T80211** **CRBSI: catheter related blood stream infection - also code specified infection**

**N189** **CRD: chronic renal disease NOS**

stage 1 N181 stage 2 N182 stage 3 N183
stage 4 N184 stage 5 N185 end stage N186
RELATED Anemia in chronic kidney disease D631

**A8100** **Creutzfeldt-Jakob disease NOS**

other A8109 variant A8101
RELATED dementia F2080 w/behavioral disturbance F0281

**N189** **CRF: chronic renal failure NOS - SEE CRD for more**

RELATED Anemia in chronic kidney disease D631

**N189** **CRI: chronic renal insufficiency - SEE CRD for more**

**K5080** **Crohn's disease both large & small intestine NOS**

w/rectal bleeding K50811
w/intestinal obstruction K50812
w/fistula K50813 w/abscess K50814
w/other complication K50818
complication NOS K50819

**K5010** **Crohn's disease large intestine NOS**

w/rectal bleeding K50111
w/intestinal obstruction K50112
w/fistula K50113 w/abscess K50114
w/other complication K50118
complication NOS K50119

**K5000** **Crohn's disease small intestine**

w/rectal bleeding K50011
w/intestinal obstruction K50012
w/fistula K50013 w/abscess K50014
w/other complication K50018
complication NOS K50019

**K5090** **Crohn's disease unspecified intestine NOS**

w/rectal bleeding K50911
w/intestinal obstruction K50912
w/fistula K50913 w/abscess K50914
w/other complication K50918
Complication NOS K50919

**R7982** **CRP: c-reactive protein elevated**

**CRPS: Complex regional pain syndrome**

CRPS I
arm: right G90511 left G90512 bilat G90513 NOS G90519
leg: right G90521 left G90522 bilat G90523 NOS G90529
other site G9059 unspecified G9050
CRPS II
leg: right G5771 left G5772 NOS G5770
arm: right G5641 left G5642 NOS G5640

**CRPS: complex regional pain syndrome SEE Pain syndrome complex regional**

**M341** **CRST: calcinosis Raynauds sclerodactyltelangiectasis also CREST**

**B459** **Cryptococcosis unspecified**

Pulmonary B450 Cerebral B451
Cutaneous B452 Osseous B453
Disseminated / Generalized B457
Other B458

**A072** **Cryptosporidiosis**

**R82998** **Crystalluria**

**G4731** **CSA: central sleep apnea primary**

in other conditions G4737

**CSF leak SEE Cerebrospinal fluid leak**

**G5600** **CTS: carpal tunnel syndrome NOS**

right G5601 left G5602 bilateral G5603

**E249** **Cushing's syndrome NOS**

pituitary dependent E240 drug induced E242
alcohol induced / pseudo E244 other E248
Nelson's syndrome E241 ectopic ACTH syndrome E243

**CVA late effect monoplegia**

unspecified side: arm I69339 leg I69349
dominant arm: right I69331 left I69332
nondominant arm: right I69333 left I69334
dominant leg: right I69341 left I69342
nondominant leg: right I69343 left I69344

**Z8673** **CVA: cerebrovascular accident - history**

**I639** **CVA: cerebrovascular accident acute/NOS (stroke)**

**R230** **Cyanosis**

**G96191** **Cyst nerve root Cervical / Lumbar / Sacral / Thoracic**

**E849** **Cystic fibrosis NOS**

w/meconium ileus E8411
other intestinal manifestations E8419
w/other manifestations E848
w/pulmonary manifestations E840
Code Also exocrine pancreatic insufficiency K8681

**A5401** **Cystitis gonococcal**

**N3090** **Cystitis NOS**

NOS w/hematuria N3091
acute: NOS N3000 w/hematuria N3001
interstitial chronic N3010 w/hematuria N3011
other chronic N3020 w/hematuria N3021
trigonitis N3030 w/hematuria N3031
irradiation N3040 w/hematuria N3041
other N3080 w/hematuria N3081

**Z435** **Cystostomy aftercare**

aftercare for other urinary tract opening Z436

**T83510-** **Cystostomy catheter infected / inflammed**

7th character indicates encounter
A - initial encounter D - subsequent encounter S - sequela
Use additional code to identify infection

**T83090-** **Cystostomy complication mechanical other**

displacement T83020- leakage T83030-
mechanical breakdown T83010-
7th character indicates encounter
A - initial encounter D - subsequent encounter S - sequela

**N99518** **Cystostomy complication other**

hemorrhage N99510 infection N99511 malfunction N99512

**Z9350** **Cystostomy status NOS**

cutaneous-vesicostomy Z9351
appendico-vesicostomy Z9352
other specified Z9359

**D89839** **Cytokine release syndrome, grade unspecified**

grade 1 D89831 grade 2 D89832
grade 3 D89833 grade 4 D89834
grade 5 D89835

**B259** **Cytomegalic virus infection NOS**

pneumonitis B250 hepatitis B251
pancreatitis B252 other B258
mononucleosis NOS B2710
mono w/polyneuropathy B2711
mono w/meningitis B271
mono w/ other complication NEC B2719

# I10 Cheat Sheet for Home Care - FY 2023

# D

**M5136** **DDD: degenerative disc disease NOS - lumbar**

thoracolumbar M5135
lumbosacral M5137
thoracic M5134

**R5381** **Debility NOS**

age related R54

**R29898** **Decline in function acute**

**DECUBITUS ULCER -- SEE pressure ulcer at site**

**Z4502** **Defibrillator fitting & adjustment implantable**

**E7081** **Deficiency Aromatic L-amino acid decarboxylase**

**E630** **Deficiency essential fatty acid**

**E619** **Deficiency nutrient element NOS**

calcium E58 selenium E59 zinc E60
copper E610 iron E611 magnesium E612

**E639** **Deficiency nutritional NOS**

**Deficiency sequelae - Code first the actual sequelae**

d/t protein-calorie malnutrition E640
d/t vitamin A deficiency E641
d/t vitamin C deficiency E642
d/t rickets, vit D deficiency E643
d/t unspecified nutrition deficiency E649
other nutritional deficiency E648

**E519** **Deficiency thiamine NOS**

dry beriberi E5111 wet beriberi E5112
Wernicke's encephalopathy E512 other E518

**E509** **Deficiency vitamin A NOS**

w/conjunctival xerosis: E500 w/Bitot's spot E501
w/corneal xerosis: E502 w/ulceration E503
w/keratomalacia E504 w/night blindness E505
w/non-ocular manifestations E508

**E539** **Deficiency vitamin B NOS**

other specified B vitamins E538
other includes biotin, folate, folic acid, pantothenic acid, B12

**D519** **Deficiency vitamin B12 RELATED ANEMIA unspecified**

d/t intrinsic factor deficiency D510
d/t malabsorption D511
transcobalamin II deficiency D512
other dietary deficiency D513
other deficiency D518

**E530** **Deficiency vitamin B2/riboflavin**

**E531** **Deficiency vitamin B6/pyridoxine**

**E54** **Deficiency vitamin C**

**E559** **Deficiency vitamin D NOS**

active rickets E550

**E560** **Deficiency vitamin E**

**E561** **Deficiency vitamin K**

**E860** **Dehydration -- Also code associated disorders of electrolyte and acid-base balance bel**

Hyperosmolality & hypernatremia (Sodium excess) E870
Hypo-osmolality & hyponatremia (Sodium deficiency) E871
Acidosis E872 Alkalosis E873
Mixed disorder of acid-base balance E874
Hyperkalemia E875 Hypokalemia E876
Electrolyte imbalance NOS E878

**F01A0** **Dementia vascular MILD NOS**

with behavioral disturbance with agitation F01A11
w/other behavioral disturbance F01A18
with psychotic disturbance F01A2
with mood disturbance F01A3 with anxiety F01A4

**F01C0** **Dementia vascular SEVERE NOS**

with behavioral disturbance with agitation F01C11
w/other behavioral disturbance F01C18
with psychotic disturbance F01C2
with mood disturbance F01C3 with anxiety F01C4

**F0150** **Dementia vascular unspecified severity NOS**

with behavioral disturbance with agitation F01511
w/other behavioral disturbance F01518
with psychotic disturbance F0152
with mood disturbance F0153 with anxiety F0154

**Z993** **Dependence on wheelchair Code cause first**

**F339** **Depressive disorder major recurrent episode NOS**

mild F330 moderate F331
severe F332 severe w/psychotic behavior F333
in remission NOS F3340
full remission F3342 partial remission F3341
recurrent brief episodes F338

**F329** **Depressive disorder major single episode NOS**

mild F320 moderate F321
severe NOS F322 severe w/psychotic behavior F323
partial or unspecified remission F324
n full remission F325
Depression/Depressive disorder unspecified /NOS F32A

**L239** **Dermatitis allergic CONTACT unspecified**

d/t metals L230 d/t cosmetics L232
d/t dyes L234 d/t food L236
d/t animal hair L2381 d/t adhesives L231
d/t drugs on skin L233 d/t other chemical products
d/t plants non-food L237 d/t other agent L2389

**L24A0** **Dermatitis contact d/t friction or contact with body fluids, unspecified**

Dermatitis contact d/t saliva L24A1
Dermatitis contact due to fecal, urinary or dual incontinence L24A2
Dermatitis contact d/t e friction or contact with other specified body fluids L24A9

**L24B0** **Dermatitis contact related to unspecified stoma or fistula**

related to digestive stoma or fistula L24B1
related to respiratory stoma or fistula L24B2
related to fecal or urinary stoma or fistula L24B3

**L219** **Dermatitis seborrheic NOS**

capitis L210 infantle L211 other L218

**L259** **Dermatitis unspecified form CONTACT unspecified**

d/t cosmetics L250 d/t drugs L251
d/t dyes L252 d/t other chemicals L253
d/t food on skin L254 d/t plants nonfood L255
d/t other agents L258

**M3300** **Dermatomyositis juvenile,organ involvement unspecified**

with respiratory involvement M3301
with myopathy M3302 without myopathy M3303
with other organ involvement M3309

**M3310** **Dermatomyositis other/adult, organ involvement unspecified**

with respiratory involvement M3311
with myopathy M3312
without myopathy / Dermatomyositis NOS M3313
with other organ involvement M3319

**M3393** **Dermatopolymyositis, unspecified without myopathy**

**DHTR: delayed hemolytic transfusion reaction**

after 24 hrs d/t Rh incompatibility T80411-
after 24 hrs d/t ABO incompatibility T80311-
at unspecified time d/t Rh incompatibility T80419-
at unspecified time d/t ABO incompatibility T80319-
7th character indicates encounter
A - initial encounter D - subsequent encounter S - sequela

**R7303** **Diabetes latent**

**R609** **Diabetes RELATED edema unspecified**

localized R600 generalized R601

**T383X5-** **Diabetes RELATED insulin and oral antidiabetic toxicity, adverse effect**

accidental/NOS T383X1- underdosing T383X6-
intentional self harm T383x2-
assault T383x3- undetermined T383x4-
7th character indicates encounter
A - initial encounter D - subsequent encounter S - sequela

**E1136** **Diabetes Type 2 w/complication cataract**

drug or chemical induced E0936
due to underlying condition E0836
Use additional code to identify DM control using:
nsulin Z794 oral antidiabetic or hypoglycemic drugs Z7984

**E1159** **Diabetes Type 2 w/complication circulatory, other**

peripheral angiopathy NOS E1151
peripheral angiopathy w/gangrene E1152
if specified drug or chemical induced, change 'E11' to 'E09'
if specified due to underlying condition change 'E11' to 'E08'
Use additional code to identify DM control using:
insulin Z794 oral antidiabetic or hypoglycemic drugs Z7984

**E1100** **Diabetes Type 2 w/complication hyperosmolarity NOS**

w/coma E1101
if specified drug or chemical induced, change 'E11' to 'E09'
if specified d/t underlying condition change 'E11' to 'E08'
Use additional code to identify DM control using:
insulin Z794 oral antidiabetic or hypoglycemic drugs Z7984

**E11649** **Diabetes Type 2 w/complication hypoglycemia NOS**

w/coma E11641
if specified drug or chemical induced, change 'E11' to 'E09'
if specified d/t underlying condition change 'E11' to 'E08'
Use additional code to identify DM control using:
insulin Z794 oral antidiabetic or hypoglycemic drugs Z7984

**E1110** **Diabetes Type 2 w/complication ketoacidosis w/o coma**

with coma E1111
if specified d/t underlying condition change 'E11' to 'E08'
if specified drug or chemical induced, change 'E11' to 'E09'
Use additional code to identify DM control using:
insulin Z794 oral antidiabetic or hypoglycemic drugs Z7984

**E1129** **Diabetes Type 2 w/complication kidney, w/other/tubular degeneration**

w/nephropathy/glomerulosclerosis E1121
w/chronic kidney disease E1122 also code CKD
if specified drug or chemical induced, change 'E11' to 'E09'
if specified d/t underlying condition change 'E11' to 'E08'
Chronic kidney disease codes:
NOS N189 stage 1 N181 stage 2 mild N182
stage 3 moderate N183 stage 4 severe N184
stage 5 N185 STAGE 6/end stage N186
For stage 6 (ESRD) also code dialysis status Z992
Use additional code to identify DM control using:
insulin Z794 oral antidiabetic or hypoglycemic drugs Z7984

**E1140** **Diabetes Type 2 w/complication neurological, neuropathy NOS**

w/mononeuropathy E1141
w/polyneuropathy / neuralgia E1142
w/autonomic polyneuropathy / gastroparesis E1143
w/amyotrophy E1144 other E1149
if specified drug or chemical induced, change 'E11' to 'E09'
if specified d/t underlying condition change 'E11' to 'E08'
Use additional code to identify control using:
insulin Z794 oral antidiabetic or hypoglycemic drugs Z7984

**Diabetes Type 2 w/complication retinopathy nonproliferative**

mild: NOS E11329- w/macular edema E11321-
moderate: NOS E11339- w/macular edema E11331-
severe: NOS E11349- w/macular edema E11341-
Designate laterality with 7th character:
right eye 1 left eye 2 bilateral 3 unspecified eye 9
if specified drug or chemical induced, change 'E11' to 'E09'
if specified d/t underlying condition change 'E11' to 'E08'
Use additional code to identify control using:
insulin Z794 oral antidiabetic or hypoglycemic drugs Z7984

**E11319** **Diabetes Type 2 w/complication retinopathy NOS**

w/macular edema E11311
if specified drug or chemical induced, change 'E11' to 'E09'
if specified due to underlying condition, change 'E11' to 'E08'
Use additional code to identify control using:
Use additional code to identify control using:
insulin Z794 oral antidiabetic or hypoglycemic drugs Z7984

**E11359** **Diabetes Type 2 w/complication retinopathy proliferative NOS**

w/macular edema E11351
if specified drug or chemical induced, change 'E11' to 'E09'
if specified due to underlying condition, change 'E11' to 'E08'
Use additional code to identify control using:
insulin Z794 oral antidiabetic or hypoglycemic drugs Z7984

| | |
|---|---|
| | **Diabetes Type 2 w/complication skin** |
| | dermatitis E11620 foot ulcer E11621<br>other skin ulcer E11622<br>other skin complication E11628<br>Also code ulcers at site<br>if specified drug or chemical induced, change 'E11' to 'E09'<br>if specified d/t underlying condition change 'E11' to 'E08'<br>Use additional code to identify control using:<br>insulin Z794 oral antidiabetic or hypoglycemic drugs Z7984 |
| **E1137x-** | **Diabetes Type 2 w/diabetic macular edema, resolved following treatment** |
| | Designate laterality with 7th character:<br>right eye 1 left eye 2 bilateral 3 unspecified eye 9<br>Use additional code to identify control using:<br>nsulin Z794 oral antidiabetic or hypoglycemic drugs Z7984<br>if specified drug or chemical induced, change 'E11' to 'E09'<br>if specified d/t underlying condition change 'E11' to 'E08' |
| **E11610** | **Diabetes Type 2 w/diabetic neuropathic arthropathy** |
| | other arthropathy E11618<br>if specified d/t underlying condition change 'E11' to 'E08'<br>if specified drug or chemical induced, change 'E11' to 'E09'<br>Use additional code to identify control using:<br>nsulin Z794 oral antidiabetic or hypoglycemic drugs Z7984 |
| **E119** | **Diabetes Type 2 w/o complication NOS** |
| | if specified d/t underlying condition change 'E11' to 'E08'<br>if specified drug or chemical induced, change 'E11' to 'E09'<br>Use additional code to identify control using:<br>insulin Z794 oral antidiabetic or hypoglycemic drugs Z7984 |
| **E11630** | **Diabetes Type 2 w/periodontal disease** |
| | other oral complication E11638<br>if specified d/t underlying condition change 'E11' to 'E08'<br>if specified drug or chemical induced, change 'E11' to 'E09'<br>Use additional code to identify control using:<br>insulin Z794 oral antidiabetic or hypoglycemic drugs Z7984 |
| **T8571x-** | **Dialysis catheter peritoneal infected/inflammed** |
| | 7th character indicates encounter<br>A - initial encounter D - subsequent encounter S - sequela<br>Use additional code to identify infection |
| **N80B39** | **Diaphragm endometriosis NOS** |
| | Superficial N80B31 Deep N80B32 |

**R197** **Diarrhea NOS**

chronic noninfectious K529
functional K591 dietetic K522
amebic A060 psychogenic F458
postproc gastrointestinal surgery k911
other postproc K9189
dysenteric/epidemic/infectious NOS A09

**D65** **DIC: disseminated intravascular coagulopathy**

**G830** **Diplegia**

**M048** **DIRA: Deficiency of interleukin 1 receptor antagonist**

**M4810** **DISH: diffuse idiopathic skeletal hyperostosis NOS**

occipito-atlanto-axial M4811
cervical M4812 cervicothoracic M4813
thoracic M4814 thoracolumbar M4815
lumbar M4816 lumbosacral M4817
sacral and sacrococcygeal M4818 multiple sites M4819

**F429** **Disorder obsessive compulsive unspecified**

Mixed obsessional thoughts and acts F422
Hoarding disorder F423
Excoriation (skin-picking) disorder F424
Other OCD F428
If appropriate may also code Obsessive-compulsive personality disorder F605

**D6959** **DIT: drug induced thrombocytopenia**

**R42** **Dizziness**

**M1990** **DJD: degenerative joint disease NOS**

**E1010** **DKA: diabetic ketoacidosis type I DM w/o coma**

w/coma E1011

**E109** **DM: diabetes mellitus type I NOS**

**E119** **DM: diabetes mellitus unspecified or type II NOS SEE diabetes for more**

**A312** **DMAC: disseminated mycobacterium avium-intracellulare complex**

**G241** **DMD: dystonia musculorum deformans**

**E11311x** **DME: diabetic macular edema (Type 2 diabetes mellitus) w/unspecified diabetic retin**

7th character indicates eye for codes below
right 1 left 2 bilateral 3 unspecified 9
w/moderate nonproliferative diabetic retinopathy E11331-
w/severe nonproliferative diabetic retinopathy E11341-
w/proliferative diabetic retinopathy E11351-
w/mild nonproliferative diabetic retinopathy E11321-

**Z66** **DNR: do not resuscitate status**

**D7212** **DRESS: Drug rash with eosinophilia and systemic symptoms syndrome**

**DRESSING CHANGE - SEE wound aftercare**

**R400** **Drowsiness**

**Z5181** **Drug level monitoring (therapeutic drug)**

Also code applicable 'drug use medical long term' (current)

**Drug resistant infection SEE infection resistant**

**Z79899** **Drug use medical long term (current) other**

aspirin Z7982 other NSAID Z791
antithrombotics/antiplatelets Z7902
antibiotics Z792 insulin Z794
hormonal contraceptives Z793
inhaled steroids Z7951 systemic steroids Z7952
bisphosphonates Z7983 anticoagulants Z7901
hypoglycemic / antidiabetic oral Z7984 injectable Z7985
Hormone replacement therapy Z79890
opiate analgesic / methadone Z79891
RELATED drug level monitoring Z5181

**R682** **Dry mouth, unspecified**

**L565** **DSAP: disseminated superficial actinic porokeratosis**

**DSTR: delayed serologic transfusion reaction**

d/t Rh incompatibility T8049x-
d/t ABO incompatibility T8039x-
unsp incompatibility T8089x -
7th character indicates encounter
A- initial encounter D- subsequent encounter S- sequela

**F10231** **DT's: delerium tremens NOS**

**K911** **Dumping syndrome**

**Duodenal ulcer SEE ULCER GI**

**K2980** **Duodenitis NOS**

w/bleeding K2981

**K317** **Duodenum polyp**

**K269** **Duodenum ulcer NOS**

acute: w/hemorrhage K260 w/perforation K261
acute: NOS K263 w/both hemorrhage /perforation K262
chronic/unsp: w/hemorrhage K264 w/perforation K265
chronic/unsp: w/both hemorrhage / perforation K266
chronic NOS K267

**Z86718** **DVT personal history of deep vein thrombosis**

**DVT: deep vein thrombosis NOS - SEE LEG THROMBOSIS for specified veins code**

ARM Acute - right I82621 left I82622
bilateral I82623 unspecified I82629
ARM Chronic - right I82721 left I82722
bilateral I82723 unspecified I82729
LEG Acute - right I82401 left I82402
bilateral I82403 unspecified I82409
LEG Chronic - right I82501 left I82502
bilateral I82503 unspecified I82509

N9410 **Dyspareunia unspecified**

Superficial (introital) N9411 Deep N9412 Other N9419

K30 **Dyspepsia functional**

I69391 **Dysphagia following cerebral infarction - Also code phase of dysphagia BELOW**

RELATED history of tobacco dependence Z87891

R1310 **Dysphagia NOS (phases)**

oral phase R1311 oropharyngeal phase R1312
pharyngeal phase R1313 pharyngoesophageal phase R1314
other / cervical / neurogenic R1319

R4702 **Dysphasia NOS**

d/t CVA or CVD I69921

R0600 **Dyspnea NOS**

orthopnea R0601 shortness of breath R0602
other forms of dyspnea R0609

G904 **Dysreflexia autonomic**

RELATED
fecal impaction K5641 urinary tract infection N390

G249 **Dystonia NOS**

idiopathic nonfamilial G242
idiopathic orofacial G244
blepharospasm NOS G245
spasmodic torticollis G243
genetic torsion G241
drug induced: subacute G2401 acute G2402 other G2409
other G248

R300 **Dysuria**

painful urination NOS R309

# I10 Cheat Sheet for Home Care - FY 2023

**EAR INFECTION - SEE OTITIS**

**Ear Perichondritis SEE Perichondritis ear external**

**H6120** **Ear wax impacted NOS**

right H6121 left H6122 bilat H6123

**H9209** **Earache NOS**

right H9201 left H9202 bilat H9203

**F509** **Eating disorder, unspecified/other specified feeding disorder**

Anorexia nervosa unspecified F5000
Anorexia nervosa, restricting type F5001
Anorexia nervosa, binge eating/purging type F5002
Bulimia nervosa F502
Binge eating disorder F5081
other/adult pica/psychogenic loss of appetite F5089
Avoidant/restrictive food intake disorder F5082

**A984** **Ebola virus disease**

**B2700** **EBV: Epstein Barr virus infection (mononucleosis) unsp**

w/meningitis B2702 w/polyneuropathy B2701
w/complication other B2709

**R233** **Ecchymoses spontaneous**

**E8889** **ECD: Erdheim-Chester disease**

**R9431** **ECG: electrocardiogram abnormal**

**Z9281** **ECMO: extracorporeal membrane oxygenation personal history**

**T783XX -** **Edema angioneurotic / allergic**

7th character indicates encounter
A - initial encounter D - subsequent encounter S - sequela

**R609** **Edema NOS**

localized NOS R600 generalized NOS R601
malignant A480 nutritional severe NOS E43
nutritional w/dyspigmentation of skin & hair E40

**Q7960** **EDS: Ehlers-Danlos syndrome unspecified**

classical (cEDS) Q7961 hypermobile (hEDS) Q7962
vascular (vEDS) Q7963 other Q7969

**R9401** **EEG: electroencephalogram abnormal NOS**

**M2540** **Effusion of joint NOS SEE site for more**

**M301** **EGPA: Eosinophilic granulomatosis with polyangiitis**

**N8502** **EIN: Endometrium intraepithelial neoplasia**

**I2783** **Eisenmenger's syndrome**

**R9431** **EKG: electrocardiogram abnormal**

**M24629** **Elbow ankylosis unspecified**
right M24621 left M24622

**M25729** **Elbow bone spur (osteophyte) unspecified**
right M25721 left M25722

**Elbow bursitis**
olecranon: unsp M7020 right M7021 left M7022
other: unsp M7030 right M7031 left M7032

**M71429** **Elbow calcification unspecified**
right M71421 left M71422

**M94229** **Elbow chondromalacia unspecified**
right M94221 left M94222

**M24529** **Elbow chondromalacia unspecified**
right M94221 left M94222

**M24529** **Elbow contractures unspecified**
right M24521 left M24522

**M25429** **Elbow effusion (joint) unspecified**
right 25421 left M25422

**Elbow gout acute / NOS**
idiopathic/primary right M10021 left M10022 unsp M10029
drug induced right M10221 left M10222 unsp M10229
d/t renal impairment right M10321 left M10322 unsp M10329
lead induced right M10121 left M10122 unsp M10129
other secondary right M10421 left M10422 unsp M10429

**Elbow gout chronic**
idiopathic/primary right M1A021- left M1A022- unsp M1A029-
lead induced right M1A121- left M1A122- unsp M1A129-
drug induced right M1A221- left M1A222- unsp M1A229-
d/t renal impairment right M1A321- left M1A322- unsp M1A329-
other secondary right M1A421- left M1A422- unsp M1A429-
The appropriate 7th character:
0 = without tophus (tophi) 1 = with tophus (tophi)

**M25029** **Elbow hemarthrosis unspecified**
right M25021 left M25022

**M24829** **Elbow joint instability NOS unspecified**
right M24821 left M24822

**M24029** **Elbow joint mice unspecified**
right M24021 left M24022

**M19029** **Elbow osteoarthritis primary unspecified**
right M19021 left M19022

**M25529** **Elbow pain NOS unspecified**

right M25521 left M25522

**Elbow ulcer pressure**

NOS: LEFT L89029 RIGHT L89019 UNSPEC L89009
unstageable: LEFT L89020 RIGHT L89010 UNSPEC L89000
stage 1: LEFT L89021 RIGHT L89011 UNSPEC L89001
stage 2: LEFT L89022 RIGHT L89012 UNSPEC L89002
stage 3: LEFT L89023 RIGHT L89013 UNSPEC L89003
stage 4: LEFT L89024 RIGHT L89014 UNSPEC L89004
LEFT pressure induced deep tissue damage L89026
RIGHT pressure induced deep tissue damage L89016
UNSPEC pressure induced deep tissue damage L89006

**Embolism and thrombosis of deep veins SEE Arm or Leg DVT**

**I423** **EMF: endomyocardial fibrosis**

**J439** **Emphysema NOS**

unilateral pulmonary J430 centrilobar J432
panlobar J431 other J438
RELATED
hx of tobacco use Z87891 tobacco use Z720
exposure to environmental smoke NOS Z7722
exposure to environmental smoke occupational Z5731

**G0400** **Encephalitis and encephalomyelitis disseminated acute NOS**

postinfectious G0401 postimmunization G0402
Encephalitis and encephalomyelitis NOS G0490

**A3981** **Encephalitis meningococcal**

**B262** **Encephalitis mumps**

**B050** **Encephalitis postmeasles**

**B0111** **Encephalitis postvaricella / postchickenpox**

**A839** **Encephalitis viral mosquito borne NOS**

Japanese A830 St Louis A833
Western equine A831 Eastern equine A832
Australian A834 California A835
Rocio virus A836

**A86** **Encephalitis viral NOS**

enteroviral A850 adenoviral A851
arthropod borne unspecified A852
lethargica A858

**B941** **Encephalitis viral SEQUELAE**

| | | |
|---|---|---|
| **A849** | **Encephalitis viral tick borne NOS** |
| | Far Eastern / Russian A840<br>Central European A841    other A841 |
| **K7682** | **Encephalopathy hepatic** |
| | Code also underlying liver disease, such as:<br>acute and subacute hepatic failure without coma K7200<br>alcoholic hepatic failure without coma K7040<br>chronic hepatic failure without coma K7210<br>hepatic failure with toxic liver disease without coma K7110<br>hepatic failure without coma K7290<br>postprocedural hepatic failure K9182 |
| **I674** | **Encephalopathy hypertensive** |
| **G0430** | **Encephalopathy necrotizing hemorrhagic acute NOS** |
| | postinfectious G0431    postimmunization G0432    other G0439 |
| **G3182** | **Encephalopathy necrotizing subacute** |
| **I6783** | **Encephalopathy syndrome posterior reversible** |
| **B376** | **Endocarditis candidal** |
| **I38** | **Endocarditis chronic NOS** |
| **I339** | **Endocarditis subacute & acute unspecified** |
| | infective I330 |
| **N72** | **Endocervicitis** |
| **N9985** | **Endometrial post ablation syndrome (PEAS)** |
| **N8040** | **Endometriosis of the rectovaginal septum, NOS** |
| | without involvement of vagina N8041<br>with involvement of vagina N8042 |
| **N808** | **Endometriosis Other not listed elsewhere** |
| **N809** | **Endometriosis unspecified (see site for more)** |
| **N719** | **Endometritis unspecified** |
| | chronic N711    acute N710 |
| **N8500** | **Endometrium hyperplasia NOS** |
| | benign / complex or simple w/o atypia N8501<br>w/atypia N8502 (EIN) |
| **N8502** | **Endometrium intraepithelial neoplasia** |
| **N840** | **Endometrium polyp** |

**A049** **Enteritis bacterial NOS**

e coli enteropathogenic A040
e coli enterotoxigenic A041
e coli enterohemorrhagic A043
e coli other A044
campylobacter A045
c. difficile A047
yersinia enterocolitica A046

**A09** **Enteritis infectious NOS**

RELATED Arthropathy M0210

**K559** **Enteritis ischemic NOS**

acute K550 chronic K551

**A084** **Enteritis viral NOS**

viral Norwalk / Norwalk like agent A0811
SRV NOS A0819 rotaviral A080
adenoviral A082 calicivirus A0831
coxsackie / echovirus / torovirus A0839
astrovirus A0832

**A047-** **Enterocolitis due to clostridium difficile**

Requires 5th character 1=recurrent 2=not specified as recurrent

**K559** **Enterocolitis NOS ischemic**

hemorrhagic acute / necrotizing NEC K550
pseudomembranous A047
staphylococcal A048
ulcerative chronic K5180
chronic K551

**K5221** **Enterocolitis syndrome food protein-induced (FPIES)**

code for hypovolemic shock, if present R571

**R94110** **EOG: electro-oculogram function study abnormal results**

**D7210** **Eosinophilia unspecified**

Familial / Hereditary D7219
Eosinophilia in diseases classified elsewhere D7218 Code first underlying disease
Drug rash with eosinophilia and systemic symptoms syndrome D7212
pulmonary eosinophilia OTHER NEC J8289
Hypereosinophilic syndrome [HES], unspecified D72119
Idiopathic hypereosinophilic syndrome [IHES] D72110
Lymphocytic Variant Hypereosinophilic Syndrome [LHES] D72111
Other hypereosinophilic syndrome D72118
Chronic/NOS eosinophilic pneumonia J8281 Acute J8282
Eosinophilic asthma J8283 Code asthma type first J45 CATEGORY

**N503** **Epididymis cyst**

**R1013** **Epigastric pain**

**J0510** **Epiglottitis acute NOS**

w/obstruction J0511

**G40909** **Epilepsy unspecified**

unsp w/status epilepticus G40901
unsp intractable G40919
unsp intractable w/status epilepticus G40911
grand mal NOS G40409
grand mal w/status epilepticus G40401
grand mal intractable G40419
grand mal intratable w/status epilepticus G40411
If applicable may also code Todds paralysis G8384
or mesial/temporal/hippocampal sclerosis G9381

**SCFE** **Epiphysis femoral capital slipped nontraumatic**

Also code for Slipped upper femoral epiphysis (SUFE)

**R040** **Epistaxis**

**R9439** **EPS: electrophysiologic studies abnormal results**

**Z171** **ER-: estrogen receptor negative status**

**Z170** **ER+: estrogen receptor positive status**

**R94111** **ERG: electroretinogram function study abnormal results**

**R142** **Eructation**

**A269** **Erysipeloid unspecified**

Erysipelothrix sepsis A267
Cutaneous A260 Other A268

**L081** **Erythrasma**

**Z1612** **ESBL: Extended spectrum beta lactamase, resistance to**

**K2090** **Esophagitis acute/NOS**

Esophagitis acute/NOS w/bleeding K2091
eosinophilic K200 reflux K210
candidiasis B3781
OTHER specified K2080 w/bleeding K2081

**K9430** **Esophagostomy complication unspecified**

hemorrhage K9431 infection K9432
malfunction K9433 other K9439

**K2080** **Esophagus abscess NOS**

**K220** **Esophagus achalasia/ aperistalsis**

**K2270** **Esophagus Barrett's**

w/ low grade dysplasia K22710
w/ high grade dysplasia K22711
w/ dysplasia, unspecified K22719

**B3781** **Esophagus candidiasis**

**K222** **Esophagus compression/obstruction incl stenosis & stricture**

**K224** **Esophagus dyskinesia/spasm**

**K2289** **Esophagus hemorrhage**

**C159** **Esophagus neoplasm malignant primary NOS**

malignant upper third C153
malignant middle third C154
malignant lower third C155
malignant overlapping sites C158
Secondary C7889 Benign D130
Mets to bone C7951 mets to unsp lymph nodes C779
mets to inguinal nodes C774 mets to axillary nodes C773
mets to esophageal nodes C771
RELATED history of tobacco dependence Z87891

**K223** **Esophagus perforation/rupture non-traumatic**

**K2281** **Esophagus polyp**

esophagogastric junction polyp K2282

**C49A1** **Esophagus stromal tumor**

**K2210** **Esophagus ulcer**

w/bleeding K2211

**I8500** **Esophagus varices NOS**

w/bleeding I8501
secondary: NOS I8510 w/bleeding I8511
FOR SECONDARY first code other disease if known

**N186** **ESRD: end stage renal disease if applicable, code first chronic hypertensive kidney**

**EAR INFECTION - SEE OTITIS**

**Ear Perichondritis SEE Perichondritis ear external**

**H6120** **Ear wax impacted NOS**

right H6121 left H6122 bilat H6123

**H9209** **Earache NOS**

right H9201 left H9202 bilat H9203

**F509** **Eating disorder, unspecified/other specified feeding disorder**

Anorexia nervosa unspecified F5000
Anorexia nervosa, restricting type F5001
Anorexia nervosa, binge eating/purging type F5002
Bulimia nervosa F502
Binge eating disorder F5081
other/adult pica/psychogenic loss of appetite F5089
Avoidant/restrictive food intake disorder F5082

**A984** **Ebola virus disease**

**B2700** **EBV: Epstein Barr virus infection (mononucleosis) unsp**

w/meningitis B2702 w/polyneuropathy B2701
w/complication other B2709

**R233** **Ecchymoses spontaneous**

**E8889** **ECD: Erdheim-Chester disease**

**R9431** **ECG: electrocardiogram abnormal**

**Z9281** **ECMO: extracorporeal membrane oxygenation personal history**

**T783XX -** **Edema angioneurotic / allergic**

7th character indicates encounter
A - initial encounter D - subsequent encounter S - sequela

**R609** **Edema NOS**

localized NOS R600 generalized NOS R601
malignant A480 nutritional severe NOS E43
nutritional w/dyspigmentation of skin & hair E40

**Q7960** **EDS: Ehlers-Danlos syndrome unspecified**

classical (cEDS) Q7961 hypermobile (hEDS) Q7962
vascular (vEDS) Q7963 other Q7969

**R9401** **EEG: electroencephalogram abnormal NOS**

**M2540** **Effusion of joint NOS SEE site for more**

**M301** **EGPA: Eosinophilic granulomatosis with polyangiitis**

**N8502** **EIN: Endometrium intraepithelial neoplasia**

**I2783** **Eisenmenger's syndrome**

**R9431** **EKG: electrocardiogram abnormal**

**M24629** **Elbow ankylosis unspecified**

right M24621 left M24622

**M25729** **Elbow bone spur (osteophyte) unspecified**

right M25721 left M25722

**Elbow bursitis**

olecranon: unsp M7020 right M7021 left M7022
other: unsp M7030 right M7031 left M7032

**M71429** **Elbow calcification unspecified**

right M71421 left M71422

**M94229** **Elbow chondromalacia unspecified**

right M94221 left M94222

**M24529** **Elbow chondromalacia unspecified**

right M94221 left M94222

**M24529** **Elbow contractures unspecified**

right M24521 left M24522

**M25429** **Elbow effusion (joint) unspecified**

right 25421 left M25422

**Elbow gout acute / NOS**

idiopathic/primary right M10021 left M10022 unsp M10029
drug induced right M10221 left M10222 unsp M10229
d/t renal impairment right M10321 left M10322 unsp M10329
lead induced right M10121 left M10122 unsp M10129
other secondary right M10421 left M10422 unsp M10429

**Elbow gout chronic**

idiopathic/primary right M1A021- left M1A022- unsp M1A029-
lead induced right M1A121- left M1A122- unsp M1A129-
drug induced right M1A221- left M1A222- unsp M1A229-
d/t renal impairment right M1A321- left M1A322- unsp M1A329-
other secondary right M1A421- left M1A422- unsp M1A429-
The appropriate 7th character:
0 = without tophus (tophi) 1 = with tophus (tophi)

**M25029** **Elbow hemarthrosis unspecified**

right M25021 left M25022

**M24829** **Elbow joint instability NOS unspecified**

right M24821 left M24822

**M24029** **Elbow joint mice unspecified**

right M24021 left M24022

**M19029** **Elbow osteoarthritis primary unspecified**

right M19021 left M19022

| | |
|---|---|
| **M25529** | **Elbow pain NOS unspecified** |
| | right M25521 left M25522 |
| | **Elbow ulcer pressure** |
| | NOS: LEFT L89029 RIGHT L89019 UNSPEC L89009 |
| | unstageable: LEFT L89020 RIGHT L89010 UNSPEC L89000 |
| | stage 1: LEFT L89021 RIGHT L89011 UNSPEC L89001 |
| | stage 2: LEFT L89022 RIGHT L89012 UNSPEC L89002 |
| | stage 3: LEFT L89023 RIGHT L89013 UNSPEC L89003 |
| | stage 4: LEFT L89024 RIGHT L89014 UNSPEC L89004 |
| | LEFT pressure induced deep tissue damage L89026 |
| | RIGHT pressure induced deep tissue damage L89016 |
| | UNSPEC pressure induced deep tissue damage L89006 |
| | **Embolism and thrombosis of deep veins SEE Arm or Leg DVT** |
| **I423** | **EMF: endomyocardial fibrosis** |
| **J439** | **Emphysema NOS** |
| | unilateral pulmonary J430 centrilobar J432 |
| | panlobar J431 other J438 |
| | RELATED |
| | hx of tobacco use Z87891 tobacco use Z720 |
| | exposure to environmental smoke NOS Z7722 |
| | exposure to environmental smoke occupational Z5731 |
| **G0400** | **Encephalitis and encephalomyelitis disseminated acute NOS** |
| | postinfectious G0401 postimmunization G0402 |
| | Encephalitis and encephalomyelitis NOS G0490 |
| **A3981** | **Encephalitis meningococcal** |
| **B262** | **Encephalitis mumps** |
| **B050** | **Encephalitis postmeasles** |
| **B0111** | **Encephalitis postvaricella / postchickenpox** |
| **A839** | **Encephalitis viral mosquito borne NOS** |
| | Japanese A830 St Louis A833 |
| | Western equine A831 Eastern equine A832 |
| | Australian A834 California A835 |
| | Rocio virus A836 |
| **A86** | **Encephalitis viral NOS** |
| | enteroviral A850 adenoviral A851 |
| | arthropod borne unspecified A852 |
| | lethargica A858 |
| **B941** | **Encephalitis viral SEQUELAE** |

**A849** **Encephalitis viral tick borne NOS**

Far Eastern / Russian A840
Central European A841 other A841

**K7682** **Encephalopathy hepatic**

Code also underlying liver disease, such as:
acute and subacute hepatic failure without coma K7200
alcoholic hepatic failure without coma K7040
chronic hepatic failure without coma K7210
hepatic failure with toxic liver disease without coma K7110
hepatic failure without coma K7290
postprocedural hepatic failure K9182

**I674** **Encephalopathy hypertensive**

**G0430** **Encephalopathy necrotizing hemorrhagic acute NOS**

postinfectious G0431 postimmunization G0432 other G0439

**G3182** **Encephalopathy necrotizing subacute**

**I6783** **Encephalopathy syndrome posterior reversible**

**B376** **Endocarditis candidal**

**I38** **Endocarditis chronic NOS**

**I339** **Endocarditis subacute & acute unspecified**

infective I330

**N72** **Endocervicitis**

**N9985** **Endometrial post ablation syndrome (PEAS)**

**N8040** **Endometriosis of the rectovaginal septum, NOS**

without involvement of vagina N8041
with involvement of vagina N8042

**N808** **Endometriosis Other not listed elsewhere**

**N809** **Endometriosis unspecified (see site for more)**

**N719** **Endometritis unspecified**

chronic N711 acute N710

**N8500** **Endometrium hyperplasia NOS**

benign / complex or simple w/o atypia N8501
w/atypia N8502 (EIN)

**N8502** **Endometrium intraepithelial neoplasia**

**N840** **Endometrium polyp**

| | | |
|---|---|
| **A049** | **Enteritis bacterial NOS** |
| | e coli enteropathogenic A040<br>e coli enterotoxigenic A041<br>e coli enterohemorrhagic A043<br>e coli other A044<br>campylobacter A045<br>c. difficile A047<br>yersinia enterocolitica A046 |
| **A09** | **Enteritis infectious NOS** |
| | RELATED Arthropathy M0210 |
| **K559** | **Enteritis ischemic NOS** |
| | acute K550 chronic K551 |
| **A084** | **Enteritis viral NOS** |
| | viral Norwalk / Norwalk like agent A0811<br>SRV NOS A0819 rotaviral A080<br>adenoviral A082 calicivirus A0831<br>coxsackie / echovirus / torovirus A0839<br>astrovirus A0832 |
| **A047-** | **Enterocolitis due to clostridium difficile** |
| | Requires 5th character 1=recurrent 2=not specified as recurrent |
| **K559** | **Enterocolitis NOS ischemic** |
| | hemorrhagic acute / necrotizing NEC K550<br>pseudomembranous A047<br>staphylococcal A048<br>ulcerative chronic K5180<br>chronic K551 |
| **K5221** | **Enterocolitis syndrome food protein-induced (FPIES)** |
| | code for hypovolemic shock, if present R571 |
| **R94110** | **EOG: electro-oculogram function study abnormal results** |
| **D7210** | **Eosinophilia unspecified** |
| | Familial / Hereditary D7219<br>Eosinophilia in diseases classified elsewhere D7218 Code first underlying disease<br>Drug rash with eosinophilia and systemic symptoms syndrome D7212<br>pulmonary eosinophilia OTHER NEC J8289<br>Hypereosinophilic syndrome [HES], unspecified D72119<br>Idiopathic hypereosinophilic syndrome [IHES] D72110<br>Lymphocytic Variant Hypereosinophilic Syndrome [LHES] D72111<br>Other hypereosinophilic syndrome D72118<br>Chronic/NOS eosinophilic pneumonia J8281 Acute J8282<br>Eosinophilic asthma J8283 Code asthma type first J45 CATEGORY |
| **N503** | **Epididymis cyst** |

**R1013** **Epigastric pain**

**J0510** **Epiglottitis acute NOS**

w/obstruction J0511

**G40909** **Epilepsy unspecified**

unsp w/status epilepticus G40901
unsp intractable G40919
unsp intractable w/status epilepticus G40911
grand mal NOS G40409
grand mal w/status epilepticus G40401
grand mal intractable G40419
grand mal intratable w/status epilepticus G40411
If applicable may also code Todds paralysis G8384
or mesial/temporal/hippocampal sclerosis G9381

**SCFE** **Epiphysis femoral capital slipped nontraumatic**

Also code for Slipped upper femoral epiphysis (SUFE)

**R040** **Epistaxis**

**R9439** **EPS: electrophysiologic studies abnormal results**

**Z171** **ER-: estrogen receptor negative status**

**Z170** **ER+: estrogen receptor positive status**

**R94111** **ERG: electroretinogram function study abnormal results**

**R142** **Eructation**

**A269** **Erysipeloid unspecified**

Erysipelothrix sepsis A267
Cutaneous A260 Other A268

**L081** **Erythrasma**

**Z1612** **ESBL: Extended spectrum beta lactamase, resistance to**

**K2090** **Esophagitis acute/NOS**

Esophagitis acute/NOS w/bleeding K2091
eosinophilic K200 reflux K210
candidiasis B3781
OTHER specified K2080 w/bleeding K2081

**K9430** **Esophagostomy complication unspecified**

hemorrhage K9431 infection K9432
malfunction K9433 other K9439

**K2080** **Esophagus abscess NOS**

**K220** **Esophagus achalasia/ aperistalsis**

**K2270** **Esophagus Barrett's**

w/ low grade dysplasia K22710
w/ high grade dysplasia K22711
w/ dysplasia, unspecified K22719

**B3781** **Esophagus candidiasis**

**K222** **Esophagus compression/obstruction incl stenosis & stricture**

**K224** **Esophagus dyskinesia/spasm**

**K2289** **Esophagus hemorrhage**

**C159** **Esophagus neoplasm malignant primary NOS**

malignant upper third C153
malignant middle third C154
malignant lower third C155
malignant overlapping sites C158
Secondary C7889 Benign D130
Mets to bone C7951 mets to unsp lymph nodes C779
mets to inguinal nodes C774 mets to axillary nodes C773
mets to esophageal nodes C771
RELATED history of tobacco dependence Z87891

**K223** **Esophagus perforation/rupture non-traumatic**

**K2281** **Esophagus polyp**

esophagogastric junction polyp K2282

**C49A1** **Esophagus stromal tumor**

**K2210** **Esophagus ulcer**

w/bleeding K2211

**I8500** **Esophagus varices NOS**

w/bleeding I8501
secondary: NOS I8510 w/bleeding I8511
FOR SECONDARY first code other disease if known

**N186** **ESRD: end stage renal disease if applicable, code first chronic hypertensive kidney**

# I10 Cheat Sheet for Home Care - FY 2023

| | |
|---|---|
| **L0201** | **Face abscess cutaneous -Does not include eye area, mouth, nose** |
| **L0203** | **Face carbuncle, code organism if known** |
| **L0202** | **Face furuncle / boil, code organism if known** |
| **G519** | **Facial nerve disorder NOS**<br>myokymia G514 palsy G510<br>clonic hemifacial spasm right G5131 left G5132<br>clonic hemifacial spasm bilat G5133 unsp G5139 |
| **R29810** | **Facial weakness / droop NOS**<br>d/t CVA I69992 |
| **R627** | **Failure to thrive (adult)** |
| **R55** | **Fainting NOS** |
| | **Fall from mobility aid**<br>powered wheelchair non-moving W050XX -<br>motorized scooter non-moving W052XX -<br>for above 7th character indicates encounter<br>A - initial encounter D - subsequent encounter S - sequela<br>mobility scooter moving V00831<br>powered wheelchair moving V00811 |
| **Z9181** | **Fall history of or at risk of**<br>repeated or tendency to fall R296 |
| **W19XXX -** | **Fall NOS**<br>from chair W07XXX -<br>from commode/toilet NOS W1811X -<br>from bed W06XXX- on ramp W102XX-<br>on stairs and steps W108XX -<br>from sidewalk curb W101XX -<br>n shower / empty bathtub W182XX -<br>in filled bathtub W16212-<br>7th character indicates encounter<br>A- initial encounter D- subsequent encounter S- sequela |
| **N7091** | **Fallopian tube abscess unspecified**<br>chronic N7011 acute/subacute N7001 |
| **N8340** | **Fallopian tube and ovary prolapse and hernia unspecified side**<br>right N8341 left N8342 |
| **N83329** | **Fallopian tube atrophy unspecified side / NOS**<br>right N83321 left N83322<br>IF ovary and fallopian tube both:<br>unspecified N8340 right N8341 left N8342 |
| **N838** | **Fallopian tube cyst** |

**N80209** **Fallopian tube endometriosis NOS**

Right unspecified N80201 superficial N80211 deep N80221
Left unspecified N80202 superficial N80212 deep N80222
Bilateral unspecified N80203 superficial N80213 deep N80223
Unspec unspecified N80209 superficial N80219 deep N80229

**N848** **Fallopian tube polyp**

**N83529** **Fallopian tube torsion unspecified side**

right N83521 left N83522
with ovary, ovarian pedicle N8353

**Family history**

sudden cardiac death Z824 stroke Z823
malignant neoplasms unsp Z809

**I743** **FAO: femoral artery occlusion**

**R5383** **Fatigue NOS**

chronic fatigue unspecified R5382 d/t senile debility R54
post viral fatigue syndrome G9331
chronic fatigue syndrome / Myalgic encephalomyelitis G9332
Other post infection and related fatigue syndromes G9339
neoplasm related (malignant) R530 Code neoplasm first
d/t excessive exertion T733xx - heat fatigue T676xx -
For codes beginning with T, 7th character indicates encounter
A - initial encounter D- subsequent encounter S- sequela

**R195** **Fecal abnormalities - color, bulk, mucus, occult blood**

**K5641** **Fecal impaction**

**R159** **Fecal incontinence NOS**

incomplete R150 smearing R151 urgency R152

**R6330** **Feeding difficulties unspecified**

Feeding problem (elderly) (infant) NOS R6339

**M0500** **Felty's syndrome NOS**

shoulder: right M05011 left M05012 unsp M05019
elbow: right M05021 left M05022 unsp M05029
wrist: right M05031 left M05032 unsp M05039
hand: right M05041 left M05042 unsp M05049
hip: right M05051 left M05052 unsp M05059
knee: right M05061 left M05062 unsp M05069
ankle & foot: right M05071 left M05072 unsp M05079
multiple sites M0509

**Femoral epiphysis slipped, upper nontraumatic**

Acute: unsp M93003 right M93011 left M93012
Chronic: unsp M93023 right M93021 left M93022
Acute on chronic: unsp M93033 right M93031 left M93032
Unsp: unsp M93003 right M93001 left 93002

**G5720** **Femoral nerve lesion unspecified lower limb**

right G5721 left G5722 bilateral G5723

**S72416-** **Femur fracture condyle NOS Unspecified CLOSED**

right S72414- left S72415-
Displaced: right S72411- left S72412- unspecified S72413-
ADD the appropriate 7th character:
A - initial encounter for closed fracture
D - subsequent encounter for closed fracture with routine healing
G - subsequent encounter for closed fracture with delayed healing
K - subsequent encounter for closed fracture with nonunion
P - subsequent encounter for closed fracture with malunion
S - sequela
For more specific change 5th character
3= medial condyle 2=lateral condyle

**S72059-** **Femur fracture head NOS Unspecified CLOSED**

right S72051- left S72052-
A - initial encounter for closed fracture
D - subsequent encounter for closed fracture with routine healing
G - subsequent encounter for closed fracture with delayed healing
K - subsequent encounter for closed fracture with nonunion
P - subsequent encounter for closed fracture with malunion
S - sequela
For shaft NOS fx change 4th /5th character to 3 0
For subcapial fx change 4th /5th character to 0 1
For trochnter NOS fx change 4th /5th character to 1 0

**M87059** **Femur osteonecrosis unspecified side**

Right M87051 left M87052

**R509** **Fever NOS**

drug induced R502 postprocedural R5082
postvaccination R5083 posttransfusion R5084
w/ conditions classified elsewhere R5081

**A8183** **FFI: fatal familial insomnia**

**M724** **Fibromatosis pseudosarcomatous**

**M797** **Fibromyalgia NOS - Code also used for fibromyositis / fibrositis / myofibrositis**

**L03019** **Finger cellulitis unspecified**

right L03011 left L03012

**Finger(s) fracture pathological NOS**

unsp M84446- right M84444- left M84445-
Change 4th character to 5 for 'in neoplastic disease'
7th character indicates encounter/status
A - initial S - sequela D - subsequent routine healing
G - subsequent delayed healing
K - subsequent nonunion P - subsequent malunion

**R143 Flatulence**

**FLU - SEE Influenza**

**E878 Fluid disorder/imbalance NOS**

**E8770 Fluid overload NOS**

d/t transfusion E8771 other E8779

**R609 Fluid retention NOS**

**I773 FMD: fibromuscular dysplasia of artery**

**R5084 FNHTR: febrile nonhemolytic transfusion reaction**

**A059 Food borne intoxication unspecified**

Staph A050 Botulism A051
Clostridium perfringens/ welchii A052
Vibrio parahaemolyticus A053
Bacillus cereus A054 Vibrio vulnificus A055
Other specified bacterial foodborne intoxications A058

**L02619 Foot abscess cutaneous unspecified**

right L02611 left L02612

**M24676 Foot ankylosis unspecified**

right M24674 left M24675

**S90829 Foot blister unspecified**

7th character indicates encounter
A- initial encounter D- subsequent encounter S- sequela

**L02629 Foot boil/ furuncle unspecified**

right L02621 left L02622

**Foot bone spur**

calcaneal NOS right M7731 left M7732 unspecified M7730
osteophyte right M25774 left M25775 unspecified M25776

**M14679 Foot Charcot's joint (and ankle) unspecified**

right M14671 left M14672

**M24576 Foot contractures unspecified**

right M24574 left M24575

**M24176 Foot crepitus (joint) unspecified**

right M24174 left M24175

**M21379** **Foot drop acquired unspecified**

right M21371 left M21372

**R601** **Foot edema NOS**

**M25476** **Foot effusion unspecified**

right M25474 left M25475

**M7750** **Foot enthesopathy unspecified (also ankle)**

Right M7751 left M7752

**Foot fracture pathological NOS**

Change 4th character to 5 for 'in neoplastic disease'
unspecified M84476- right M84474- left M84475-
7th character indicates encounter/status
A - initia S - sequela
D - subsequent routine healing
G - subsequent delayed healing
K - subsequent nonunion P - subsequent malunion
For fracture w/osteoporosis, see Foot osteoporosis

**Foot gout acute/NOS (and ankle, toe)**

idiopathic/primary right M10071 left M10072 unsp M10079
lead induced right M10171 left M10172 unsp M10179
drug induced right M10271 left M10272 unsp M10279
d/t renal impairment right M10371 left M10372 unsp M10379
other secondary right M10471 left M10472 unsp M10479

**Foot gout chronic (also ankle, toe)**

idiopathic/primary right M1A071- left M1A072- unsp M1A079-
lead induced right M1A171- left M1A172- unsp M1A179-
drug induced right M1A271- left M1A272- unsp M1A279-
d/t renal impairment right M1A371- left M1A372- unsp M1A379-
other secondary right M1A471- left M1A472- unsp M1A479-
ADD The appropriate 7th character:
0 = without tophus (tophi) 1 = with tophus (tophi)

**M25076** **Foot hemarthrosis unspecified**

right M25074 left M25075

**M9279** **Foot joints chondromalacia unspecified**

right M94271 left M94272

**M19079** **Foot osteoarthritis (& ankle) primary unspecified**

right M19071 left M19072

**Foot osteomyelitis NOS**

acute hematogenous: right M86071 left M86072 unsp M86079
acute other: right M86171 left M86172 unsp M86179
subacute: right M86271 left M86272 unsp M86279
chronic multifocal: right M86371 left M86372 unsp M86379
chronic draining: right M86471 left M86472 unsp M86479
chronic hematogenous: right M86571 left M86572 unsp M86579
chronic other: right M86671 left M86672 unsp M86679

**Foot osteonecrosis**

idiopathic: right M87074 left M87075 unsp M87076
d/t drugs: right M87174 left M87175 unsp M87176
d/t trauma: right M87274 left M87275 unsp M87276
other secondary: right M87374 left M87375 unsp M87376
other: right M87874 left M87875 unsp M87876

**M80079- Foot osteoporosis age related w/current fracture unspecified**

right M80071- left M80072-
7th character indicates encounter/status
A - initial D - subsequent routine healing
G - subsequent delayed healing P - subsequent malunion
K - subsequent nonunion S - sequela

**M25579 Foot pain unspecified**

right M25571 left M25572

**Foot tendon rupture NOS non-traumatic / spontaneous**

extensor: right M66271 left M66272 unsp M66279
flexor: right M66371 left M66372 unsp M66379
other: right M66871 left M66872 unsp M66879

**L97509 Foot ulcer other part non-pressure chronic UNSPECIFIED side NOS**

ncludes toe; SEE HEEL for midfoot & heel
for RIGHT SIDE change 5th character to 1
for LEFT SIDE change 5th character to 2
limited to skin L97501 w/fat layer exposed L97502
w/muscle necrosis L97503 w/bone necrosis L97504
w/muscle involvement without necrosis L97505
w/bone involvement without necrosis L97506
with other specified severity L97508

**K5221 FPIES - Food protein-induced enterocolitis syndrome**

**E7800 Fredrickson's hyperlipoproteinemia type IIa**

**R627 FTT: failure to thrive adult**

**R509 FUO: fever of unknown origin NOS**

# G

**D550** **G-6-PD: anemia of G-6-PD (includes G6pd deficiency)**

**F411** **GAD: generalized anxiety disorder**

**K810** **Gallbladder abscess/empyema/gangrene NOS**

**K8060** **Gallbladder calculus and bile duct calculus w/cholecystitis NOS**

NOS w/obstruction K8061
w/acute cholecystitis K8062 w/obstruction K8063
w/chronic cholecystitis K8064 w/obstruction K8065
w/acute & chronic cholecystitis K8066 w/obstruction K8067

**K824** **Gallbladder cholesterolosis / strawberry**

**K829** **Gallbladder disease NOS**

Also use this code for adhesions/atrophy/cyst/hypertrophy/ulcer

**K823** **Gallbladder fistula**

**K821** **Gallbladder hydrops / mucocele**

**K820** **Gallbladder obstruction/occlusion/stenosis w/o cholelithiasis**

**K822** **Gallbladder perforation**

**K563** **Gallstone ileus**

**K8020** **Gallstone impacted / NOS**

impacted w/obstruction K8021

**I96** **Gangrene cutaneous/ dry/ extremities/ moist/ spreading**

gas A480 presenile I73 pulmonary J850
Type 2 diabetes w/diabetic gangrene E1152

**R141** **Gas pain**

**B950** **GAS: group A streptococcal disease (as cause of other disease)**

**K314** **Gastric diverticulum**

**K316** **Gastric duodenal fistula**

**K30** **Gastric hyperacidity**

**K31A29** **Gastric intestinal metaplasia with dysplasia, unspecified**

with low grade dysplasia K31A21
with high grade dysplasia K31A22

**K31A19** **Gastric intestinal metaplasia without dysplasia, unspecified site**

without dysplasia, involving the antrum K31A11
without dysplasia, involving the body K31A12
without dysplasia, involving the fundus K31A13
without dysplasia, involving the cardia K31A14
without dysplasia, involving multiple sites K31A15

**K31A0** **Gastric intestinal metaplasia, unspecified / NOS**

**K3189** **Gastric mucosa intestinal metaplasia**

**K2960** **Gastric mucosal hypertrophy**

w/ bleeding K2961

**K311** **Gastric outlet obstruction**

**K317** **Gastric polyp**

**K3189** **Gastric prolapse/rupture**

**K219** **Gastric reflux**

**K259** **Gastric ulcer NOS**

acute: w/hemorrhage K250 w/perforation K251
acute: NOS K253 w/both hemorrhage/perforation K252
chronic/unsp: w/hemorrhage K254 w/perforation K255
chronic/unsp w/both hemorrhage/perforation K256
chronic NOS K257

**F458** **Gastritis nervous/psychogenic**

**K2970** **Gastritis NOS**

NOS w/hemorrhage K2971
acute: K2900 w/hemorrhage K2901
alcoholic: K2920 w/hemorrhage K2921
chronic: K2950 w/hemorrhage K2951
chronic atrophic: K2940 w/hemorrhage K2941
chronic superficial: K2930 w/hemorrhage K2931
other: K2960 other w/hemorrhage K2961

**K2990** **Gastroduodenitis NOS**

w/bleeding K2991

**K529** **Gastroenteritis non-infective NOS**

granulomatous/regional/transmural K5010 (Crohn's)
Food protein-induced enterocolitis syndrome K5221
Food protein-induced enteropathy K5222
Other allergic and dietetic K5229
d/t radiation K520 eosinophilic K5281 Other K589

**Z4659** **Gastrointestinal appliance fitting & adjustment**

**K922** **Gastrointestinal bleeding/hemorrhage NOS**

**K9281** **Gastrointestinal mucositis ulcerative**

**C49A0** **Gastrointestinal stromal tumor unspecified**

esophagus C49A1 stomach C49A
small intestine C49A3 large intestine C49A4
rectum C49A5 other specified sites C49A9

**K289** **Gastrojejunal ulcer NOS**

acute: w/hemorrhage K280 w/perforation K281
acute: NOS K283 w/both hemorrhage/perforation K282
chronic/unsp: w/hemorrhage K284 w/perforation K285
chronic/ unspec: w/ both hemorrhage and perforation K286
chronic NOS K287

**K3184** **Gastroparesis**

**Z431** **Gastrostomy care / aftercare**

status w/o need for care Z93
fitting & adjust Z4659

**K9420** **Gastrostomy complication NOS**

hemorrhage K9421 other K9429
malfunction K9423 Infection K9422
for infection also code type eg. abd wall cellulitis L03311 or a sepsis

**B951** **GBS: group B streptococcal disease (as cause of other disease)**

**G610** **GBS: Guillain-Barre' Syndrome - also code sequelae if present G650**

**Genital herpes SEE Herpes simplex Anogenita**

**L293** **Genital itch**

**N819** **Genital prolapse female unspecified**

uterovaginal: NOS N814 complete N813 incomplete N812
urethrocele N810 rectocele N816
cystocele: NOS N8110 lateral N8112 midline N8111
vaginal enterocele N815 perineocele N8181
cervical stump N8185 pelvic muscle wasting N8184
ncompetence of pubocervical tissue N8182
incompetence of rectovaginal tissue N8183
other N8189

**K219** **GERD: gastroesophageal reflux disease NOS**

w/esophagitis K2100 w/esophagitis bleeding K2101

**A071** **Giardiasis**

**K06020** **Gingival recession generalized NOS**

minimal K06021 moderate K06022 severe K06023

**K06010** **Gingival recession localized NOS**

minimal K06011 moderate K06012 severe K06023

**A691** **Gingivitis Vincent's**

**H44519** **Glaucoma absolute**

right H44511 left H44512 bilateral H44513
See tables in back of book for more GLAUCOMA

**R7309** **Glucose abnormal NOS aka latent diabetes, pre-diabetes**

**R7301** **Glucose fasting elevated/impaired**

**R7302** **Glucose tolerance elevated/impaired (oral)**

**E74819** **Glucose transport disorder unspecified**

Glucose transporter protein type 1 deficiency E74810
Other disorders of glucose transport E74818

**D75A** **Glucose-6-phosphate dehydrogenase deficiency Do not use with D550**

**E7400** **Glycogen storage disease NOS**

type 1 E7401 (von Gierke disease)
type 2 E7402 (Pompe disease)
type 3 E7403 (Cori disease)
type 5 E7404 (McArdle disease)
other E7409
RELATED cardiomyopathy I43

**E74818** **Glycosuria Familial / renal**

**E049** **Goiter NOS**

cystic NOS / nontoxic multinodular E042
nontoxic: uninodular E041 diffuse/simple E040
toxic: nodular E0520 w/crisis E0521
iodine deficiency: diffuse E010 multinodular E011
iodine deficiency unspecified / endemic E012
dyshormogenetic E071

**A549** **Gonococcal infection unspecified**

cystitis and urethritis unsp A5401 cervicitis unsp A5403
kidney and ureter A5421 prostatitis A5422
other male genital A5423 female PID A5424
conjunctivitis A5431 keratitis A5433
spondylopathy A5441 arthritis A5442
pharyngitis A545 infection of anus & rectum A546
pneumonia A5484 sepsis A5486
This list is not all inclusive

**I43** **Gout cardiomyopathy**

**M100** **Gout NOS**

SEE Gout at foot, hand, hip, knee, elbow, toe, shoulder, wrist

**M3130** **Granulomatosis respiratory necrotizing NOS**

w/renal involvement M3131

**E0500** **Grave's disease NOS**

w/ crisis E0501

**A8182** **GSS: Gerstmann-Straussler-Scheinker syndrome**

**R7309** **GTT: glucose tolerance test oral abnormal results (non-fasting)**

**G610** **Guillain-Barre syndrome**

also code sequelae if present G650

# I10 Cheat Sheet for Home Care - FY 2023

# H

**H&M: hematemesis and melena**

hematemesis K920    melena K921

**Hallux disorders**

varus acquired unsp M2030   right M2031   left M2032
malleus acquired unsp M2040   right M2041   left M2042
rigidus acquired unsp M2020   right M2021   left M2022
valgus acquired unsp M2010   right M2011   left M2012

**Hand bone cyst**

solitary cyst: unsp M85449   right M85441   left M85442
aneurysmal cyst: change 4th digit to 5
other cyst: change 4th digit to 6

M7010 **Hand bursitis unspecified**

right M7011   left M7012

M71449 **Hand calcification unspecified**

right M71441   left M71442

M9249 **Hand chondromalacia unspecified**

right M94241   left M94242

M84443- **Hand fracture pathological NOS unspecified**

Change 4th character to 5 for 'in neoplastic disease'
right M84441-   left M84442-
7th character indicates encounter/status
A - initial   S - sequela
D - subsequent routine healing
G - subsequent delayed healing
K - subsequent nonunion   P - subsequent malunion

**Hand gout acute / NOS**

idiopathic/primary: right M10041   left M10042   unsp M10049
drug induced: right M10241   left M10242   unsp M10249
d/t renal impairment: right M10341   left M10342   unsp M10349
lead induced: right M10141   left M10142   unsp M10149
other secondary: right M10441   left M10442   unsp M10449

**Hand gout chronic**

idiopathic/primary: right M1A041-   left M1A042-   unsp M1A049-
lead induced: right M1A141-   left M1A142-   unsp M1A149-
drug induced: right M1A241-   left M1A242-   unsp M1A249-
d/t renal impairment: right M1A341-   left M1A342-   unsp M1A349-
other secondary: right M1A441-   left M1A442-   unsp M1A449-
ADD The appropriate 7th character
0 = without tophus (tophi)   1 = with tophus (tophi)

M25049 **Hand hemarthrosis unspecified**

right M19041   left M19042

**M19049** **Hand osteoarthritis primary unspecified**

right M19041 left M19042

**M80049-** **Hand osteoporosis age related w/current fracture unspecified**

right M80041- left M80042-
7th character indicates encounter/status
A - initial D - subsequent routine healing
G - subsequent delayed healing S - sequela
K - subsequent nonunion P - subsequent malunion

**A985** **Hanta virus disease with renal syndrome**

Hanta virus (cardio)-pulmonary syndrome B334

**G4732** **HAPB: high altitude periodic breathing**

**B334** **HCPS: Hantavirus cardio-pulmonary syndrome - also HPS**

**I119** **HCVD: hypertensive cardiovascular disease NOS**

w/heart failure I110 Also code heart failure
RELATED
exposure to environmental tobacco smoke Z7722
history of tobacco dependence Z87891
occupational exposure to environmental tobacco smoke Z5731
tobacco use Z720
Nicotine dependence NOS F17209 SEE Nicotine dependence for more

**L89819** **Head ulcer pressure unspecified (includes face)**

L89810 unstageable stage 1 L89811
stage 2 L89812 stage 3 L89813 stage 4 L89814
pressure-induced deep tissue damage L89816

**G44009** **Headache Cluster NOS**

ntractable G44001
episodic: NOS G44019 intractable G44011
chronic: NOS G44029 intractable G44021

**G4440** **Headache drug induced NEC NOS**

intractable G4441

**R519** **Headache NOS SEE migraine if so specified**

with orthostatic component NEC R51O

**Headache other specified**

primary thunderclap G4453
primary cough G4483 hypnic G4481
primary exertional G4484 primary stabbing G4485
new daily persistent G4452
cervicogenic G4486 Code also associated cervical spinal condition, if known

**G44309** **Headache Post-traumatic NOS**

NOS intractable G44301
acute: NOS G44319 intractale G44311
chronic: NOS G44329 intractable G44321

**G43C0** **Headache syndrome periodic NOS**

intractable G43C

**G44209** **Headache Tension NOS**

intractable G44201
episodic: NOS G44219 intractable G44211
chronic: NOS G44229 intractable G44221

**G441** **Headache vascular NEC**

**R009** **Heart beat abnormalities NOS/unspecified**

Bradycardia R001 Tachycardia R000
Palpitations R002 Other R008

**I447** **Heart block left bundle branch NOS**

left bundle branch hemi NOS I4460
left anterior fascicular I444
left posterior fascicular I445

**I459** **Heart block NOS**

bundle branch NOS I454 sinoatrial I455
bifascicular I452 trifascicular I453
AV NOS I4430 AV 1st degree I440
AV 2nd degree I441 AV 3rd degree / complete I442
AV other I4439

**I4510** **Heart block right bundle branch NOS**

right fascicular I450 right other I4519

**I119** **Heart disease hypertensive NOS**

w/heart failure I110 also code heart failure
RELATED
exposure to environmental tobacco smoke Z7722
history of tobacco dependence Z87891
occupational exposure to environmental tobacco smoke Z5731
Nicotine dependence NOS F17209 SEE Nicotine dependence for more
tobacco use Z720

**Heart disease hypertensive w/ chronic kidney disease**

w/o heart failure W/ CKD stages 1-4 or unsp I1310
w/o heart failure w/CKD stage 5 (ESRD) I1311
w/heart failure W/ CKD stages 1-4 or unsp I130
w/heart failure w/CKD stage 5 (ESRD) I132
RELATED Chronic kidney disease --
stage 1 N181 stage 2 N182 stage 3 N183
stage 4 N184 stage 5 N185 end stage N186

**I259** **Heart disease ischemic chronic/ NOS**

RELATED history of tobacco dependence Z87891

**Heart disease rheumatic acute**

pericarditis I010 endocarditis I011
myocarditis I012 other spec I018
unspecified / carditis I019

**I069** **Heart disease rheumatic chronic AORTIC VALVE unspecified**

stenosis I060 insufficiency I061
stenosis w/insufficiency I062
other specified I068

**I059** **Heart disease rheumatic chronic MITRAL VALVE unspecified**

stenosis I050 insufficiency I051
stenosis w/insufficiency I052
other specified I058

**I089** **Heart disease rheumatic chronic MULTIPLE VALVE unspecified**

mitral & aortic NOS I080
mitral & triscupid NOS I081
aortic & tricuspid NOS I082
mitral & aortic & tricuspid NOS I083
other NOS I088

**I079** **Heart disease rheumatic chronic TRICUSPID VALVE unspecified**

stenosis I070 insufficiency I071
stenosis w/insufficiency I072 other specified I078

**I099** **Heart disease rheumatic unspecified**

myocarditis I090 endocarditis I091
chronic pericarditis I092 heart failure I0981
other specified I0989

**I499** **Heart dysrhythmia NOS**

**I517** **Heart enlarged**

**I509** **Heart failure unspecified /congestive NOS**

systolic: acute I5021 chronic I5022
systolic: acute on chronic I5023 unsp I5020
diastolic: acute I5031 chronic I5032
diastolic: acute on chronic I5033 unsp I5030
combined systolic-diastolic: acute I5041 chronic I5042
combined systolic-diastolic: acute on chronic I5043 unsp I5040
postop cardiac surgery I97130
postop other surgery I97131
RELATED fluid overload E8770

**R002** **Heart palpitations**

**Heart valve disorders nonrheumatic**

PULMONARY unsp I379 other I378 stenosis I370
insufficiency I371 stenosis w/insufficiency I372
TRICUSPID unsp I369 other I368 stenosis I360
insufficiency I361 stenosis w/insufficiency I362
AORTIC unsp I359 other I358 stenosis I350
insufficiency I351 stenosis w/insufficiency I352
MITRAL unsp I349 other I348 stenosis I340
insufficiency I341 stenosis w/insufficiency I342

**R12** **Heartburn**

**T6701** **Heatstroke and sunstroke - heat apoplexy/pyrexia, siriasis, thermoplegia**

exertional T6702 other T6709

**L97409** **Heel / midfoot ulcer non-pressure chronic UNSPECIFIED side NOS**

limited to skin L97401 w/muscle necrosis L97403
w/muscle necrosis L97403 w/bone necrosis L97404
w/muscle involvement without necrosis L97405
w/bone involvement without necrosis L97406
w/ other specified severity L97408

**L97429** **Heel /midfootl ulcer non-pressure chronic LEFT NOS**

limited to skin: L97421 fat layer exposed: L97422
muscle necrosis: L97423 bone necrosis: L97424
w/muscle involvement without necrosis L97425
w/bone involvement without necrosis L97426
w/ other specified severity L97428

**L89629** **Heel ulcer pressure left NOS**

unstageable: Left L89620 Right L89610 Unspec L89600
stage 1 Left L89621 Right L89611 Unspec L89601
stage 2 Left L89622 Right 2 L89612 Unspec L89602
stage 3 Left L89623 Right L89613 Unspec L89603
stage 4 Left L89624 Right L89614 Unspec L89604
Right pressure-induced deep tissue damage L89616
Left pressure-induced deep tissue damage L89626
Unspec pressure-induced deep tissue damage L89606

**L89619** **Heel ulcer pressure right NOS**

unstageable L89610 stage 1 L89611
stage 2 L89612 stage 3 L89613 stage 4 L89614
pressure-induced deep tissue damage L89616

**L97419** **Heel/ midfoot ulcer non-pressure chronic RIGHT NOS**

limited to skin L97411 w/fat layer exposed L97412
w/muscle necrosis L97413 w/bone necrosis L97414
w/muscle involvement without necrosis L97415
w/bone involvement without necrosis L97416
w/ other specified severity L97418
For Left change 5th character to 2
For Unspecified change 5th character to 0

**M2500** **Hemarthrosis NOS**

**K920** **Hematemesis**

**K921** **Hematochezia**

**R710** **Hematocrit precipitous drop (or hemoglobin)**

**M7981** **Hematoma soft tissue nontraumatic - SEE Postop also**

**N857** **Hematometra**

**N836** **Hematosalpinx**

w/hematometra N857

**R319** **Hematuria NOS**

gross R310
benign essential microscopic R311
asymptomatic microscopic R3121
other microscopic R3129
Urinary diagnoses often have specific codes for hematuria

**N029** **Hematuria recurrent and persistent**

w/minor glomerular abnormality N020
w/focal & segmental glomerular lesions N021
w/diffuse membranous glomerulonephritis N022
w/diffuse mesangial proliferative glomerulonephritis N023
w/diffuse endocapillary proliferative glomerulonephritis N024
w/diffuse mesangiocapillary glomerulonephritis N025
w/dense deposit disease N026
w/diffuse crescentic glomerulonephritis N027
w/other morphologic changes N028
w/ C3 glomerulonephritis N02A

**G8100** **Hemiplegia & hemiparesis Flaccid NOS**

dominant side right G8101 left G8102
nondominant right G8103 left G8104

**G8190** **Hemiplegia & hemiparesis NOS**

dominant side right G8191 left G8192
nondominant right G8193 left G8194

| | |
|---|---|
| **G8110** | **Hemiplegia & hemiparesis Spastic** |
| | dominant side right G8111 left G8112<br>nondominant right G8113 left G8114 |
| **E83119** | **Hemochromatosis unspecified** |
| | d/t repeated red blood cell tranfusions E83111<br>hereditary E83110 other E83118 |
| **D5930** | **Hemolytic-uremic syndrome NOS** |
| | hemolytic-uremic syndrome infection associated D5931<br>hemolytic-uremic syndrome hereditary D5932<br>hemolytic-uremic syndrome other D5939 |
| **D66** | **Hemophilia A / NOS** |
| | hemophilia B D67 hemophilia C D681 vascular D680 |
| **R042** | **Hemoptysis** |
| **D6832** | **Hemorrhage anticoagulant induced** |
| **N950** | **Hemorrhage postmenopausal** |
| **K649** | **Hemorrhoids NOS (bleeding)** |
| | stage 1 K640 bleed w/o prolapse<br>stage 2 K641 bleed/ prolapse w/strain, then retract<br>stage 3 K642 bleed/ prolapse, require manual replace<br>stage 4 K643 bleed/ prolapse, cannot replace manually<br>K644 external NOS/ perianal venous thrombosis<br>K645 external thrombosed<br>K648 other |
| | **Hepatic - SEE also Liver** |
| **K7291** | **Hepatic coma NOS** |
| **B159** | **Hepatitis A viral acute NOS** |
| | w/hepatic coma B150 |
| **K7010** | **Hepatitis alcoholic NOS** |
| | w/ascites K7011 |
| **K754** | **Hepatitis autoimmune / Lupoid NEC** |
| **B169** | **Hepatitis B viral acute NOS** |
| | w/hepatic coma B162<br>w/delta agent NOS B161<br>w/delta agent w/hepatic coma B160 |
| **K753** | **Hepatitis granulomatous NEC** |
| **K752** | **Hepatitis nonspecific reactive** |

**B179** **Hepatitis viral NOS acute**

acute delta super infectiion of B carrier B170
hepatitis C NOS B1710
hepatits C w/hepatic coma B1711
hepatitis E acute B172
other specified NEC B178

**B189** **Hepatitis viral NOS chronic**

hepatitis NOS B B181 w/delta agent B180
hepatitis C B182
other chronic B188
These codes include: Carrier of viral hepatitis

**B942** **Hepatitis viral SEQUELAE**

**B199** **Hepatitis viral unspecified NOS**

NOS w/coma B190
B NOS B1910 B NOS w/coma B1911
C NOS B1920 C NOS w/coma B1921

**A609** **Herpes simplex infection ANOGENITAL NOS**

penis A6001 other male genital A6002
cervicitis A6003
vulvovaginitis / vulva / vagina A6004
other urogenital tract A6009
perianal skin and rectum A601
urogenital system, unspecified A6000

**B009** **Herpes simplex infection NOS**

eczema herpeticum B000 meningitis B003
vesicular dermatitis B001 encephalitis B004
gingivostomatitis /pharyngitis B002
disseminated /sepsis B007
hepatitis B0081 yelitis B0082
other/ whitlow B0089
ocular NOS B0050 iridocyclitis/ uveitis B0051
keratitis B0052 conjunctivitis B0053
other ocular B0059

**B029** **Herpes zoster NOS**

w/myelitis B0224 polyneuropathy B0223
geniculate B0221 conjunctivitis B0231
iridocyclitis B0232 scleritis B0234
keratoconjunctivitis B0233 meningitis B021
opthalmicus B0239 encephalitis B020
disseminated B027 w/other complications B028

**B084** **HFMD: hand foot mouth disease**

**E791** **HG-PRT: hypoxanthine-guanine-phosphoribosyl transferase deficiency**

**HGSIL: high grade squamous intraepithelial lesion**

from vaginal pap smear: R87623
from cervix pap smear: R87613

Q8719 **HHHO: hypotonia, hypomentia, hypogonadism, obesity syndrome**

K449 **Hiatel hernia NOS**

incarcerated/ irreducible/ obstructive/ strangulated K440
w/gangrene K441

S70219 **Hip abrasion NOS unspecified side**

right S70211- left S70212-
7th character indicates encounter
A - initial encounter D - subsequent encounter S - sequela

M24659 **Hip ankylosis unspecified**

right M24651 left M24652

**Hip arthritis NOS**

allergic/ climacteric: unsp M13859 right M13851 left M13852
crystal NOS: unsp M11859 right M11851 left M11852
degenerative: SEE hip osteoarthritis
transient: unsp M12859 right M12851 left M12852
traumatic: unsp M12559 right M12551 left M12552

M25759 **Hip bone spur (osteophyte) unspecified**

right M25751 left M25752

**Hip bursitis**

trochanteric: unsp M7060 right M7061 left M7062
other: unsp M7070 right M7071 left J7072

M71459 **Hip calcification unspecified**

right M71451 left M71452

M9259 **Hip chondromalacia unspecified**

right M94251 left M94252

M24559 **Hip contractures unspecified**

right M24551 left M24552

**Hip dislocation**

NOS: unsp S73006- right S73004- left S73005
posterior: unsp S73016- right S73014- left S73015
central: unsp S73046- right S73044- left S73045
obturator: unsp S73026- right S73024- left S73025
other anterior: NOS S73036- right S73034- left S73035
7th character indicates encounter
A - initial encounter D - subsequent encounter S - sequela

M24459 **Hip dislocation recurrent unspecified**

right M24451 left M24452

**Hip fixation internal infected**

right T84620- left T84621
7th character indicates encounter
A - initial encounter D - subsequent encounter S - sequela

**S72009-** **Hip Fracture NOS (unspecified part of neck of femur) CLOSED**

right S72001- left S72002
Add the appropriate 7th character:
A - initial encounter for closed fracture
D - subsequent encounter for closed fracture with routine healing
G - subsequent encounter for closed fracture with delayed healing
K - subsequent encounter for closed fracture with nonunion
P - subsequent encounter for closed fracture with malunion
S - sequela

**Hip gout acute/NOS**

idiopathic/primary right M10051 left M10052 unsp M10059
lead induced right M10151 left M10152 unsp M10159
drug induced right M10251 left M10252 unsp M10259
d/t renal impairment right M10351 left M10352 unsp M10359
other secondary right M10451 left M10452 unsp M10459

**Hip gout chronic**

idiopathic/primary right M1A051- left M1A052- unsp M1A059-
lead induced right M1A151- left M1A152- unsp M1A159-
drug induced right M1A251- left M1A252- unsp M1A259-
d/t renal impairment right M1A351- left M1A352- unsp M1A359-
other secondary right M1A451- left M1A452- unsp M1A459-
Add the appropriate 7th character
0 = without tophus (tophi) 1 = with tophus (tophi)

**M25059** **Hip hemarthrosis unspecified**

right M25051 left M25052

**Hip injuries superficial**

Contusion unsp S7000x- right S7001x- left S7002x-
Abrasion unsp S70219- right S70211- left S70212-
Blister (nonthermal) unsp S70221- right S70222- left S70229-
Insect bite (nonvenomous) unsp S70269- right S70261- left S70262-
7th character indicates encounter
A- initial encounter D- subsequent encounter S- sequela

**M24859** **Hip joint instability NOS unspecified**

right M4851 left M24852

**M24059** **Hip joint mice unspecified**

right M24051 left M24052

**M169** **Hip osteoarthritis NOS**

Primary: bilateral M160 unsp M1610 right M1611 left M1612
Dysplasic: bilateral M162 unsp M1630 right M1631 Left M1632
post trauma: bilateral M164 unsp M1650 right M1651 left M1652
other bilateral: M166 other unilateral: M167

**M87059** **Hip osteonecrosis idiopathic aseptic NOS**

**M80059-** **Hip osteoporosis w/current pathological fracture unspecified**

right M80051- left M80052-
7th character indicates encounter/status
A - initial
D - subsequent routine healing
G - subsequent delayed healing
K - subsequent nonunion
P - subsequent malunion
S - sequela

**M25559** **Hip pain unspecified**

right M25551 left M25552

**Z96649** **Hip replacement status NOS**

right Z96641 left Z96642 bilat Z96643

**Hip ulcer pressure contiguous site of back, buttock & hip SEE BACK ulcer pressure**

**L89229** **Hip ulcer pressure left NOS**

unstageable L89220 stage 1 L89221 stage 2 L89222
stage 3 L89223 stage 4 L89224
pressure-induced deep tissue damage L89226

**L89219** **Hip ulcer pressure right NOS**

unstageable L89210 stage 1 L89211 stage 2 L89212
stage 3 L89213 stage 4 L89214
pressure-induced deep tissue damage L89216

**L89209** **Hip ulcer pressure unspecified side NOS**

unstageable L89200 stage 1 L89201 stage 2 L89202
stage 3 L89203 stage 4 L89204
pressure-induced deep tissue damage L89206

**B399** **Histoplasmosis unspecified**

pulmonary: Acute B390 Chronic B391 unspecified B392
Disseminated / Generalized B393
American histoplasmosis unspecified B394
African histoplasmosis (duboisii) B395
RELATED
AIDS B20 Code first
Meningitis in other infectious diseases G02
Chorioretinal disorders in diseases classified elsewhere H32
Pericarditis in diseases classified elsewhere I32
Endocarditis & heart valve disorders in diseases classified elsewhere I39

**D75829** **HIT: heparin induced thrombocytopenia unspecified**

heparin induced thrombocytopenia non-immune D75821
heparin induced thrombocytopenia immune mediated D75822
heparin induced thrombocytopenia (syndrome) other D75828
heparin induced thrombocytopenia w/o heparin D7584

**HIV**

B9735 HIV 2: human immunodeficiency virus type 2 infection - used as cause of other di

Z717 HIV counseling
Z21 HIV infection asymptomatic status / HIV positive NOS
R75 HIV serologic evidence inconclusive
B20 HIV: human immunodeficiency virus infection NOS / AIDS

**L509** **Hives NOS**

**D751** **HOA: high oxygen affinity hemoglobin polycythemia, secondary polycythemia**

**C8100** **Hodgkin lymphoma nodular unspecified**

head/face/neck C8101 intrathoracic C8102 extranodal C8109
intra-abdominal C8103 axilla/arm C8104 inguinal/leg C8105
intrapelvic C8106 spleen C8107 multiple C8108
For other type Hodgkin, change 4th character:
1 = Nodular sclerosis 2 = Mixed cellularity
3 = Lymphocyte depleted 4 = Lymphocyte rich
7 = other / classical 9 = unspecified
RELATED
Personal hx of Hodgkin lymphoma Z8571

**H9190** **HOH: hard of hearing unspecified / deaf NOS**

right ear H9191 left ear H9192 bilateral H9193

**B769** **Hookworm NOS**

ancylostomiasis B760
necatoriasis B761 other B768

**K6131** **Horseshoe abscess (Ischiorectal)**

**Z515** **Hospice care, terminal care, palliative care**

**M8940** **HPOA: hypertrophic pulmonary osteoarthropathy NOS**

**Z1151** **HPV screening: human papilloma virus screening**

**A630** **HPV: human papillomavirus infection (anogenital warts)**

**R162** **HSM: hepatosplenomegaly NOS**

**B0082** **HSM: herpes simplex myelitis**

**D690** **HSP: Henoch-Schonlein purpura (allergic)**

**B009** **HSV: herpes simplex virus infection NOS**

**B9733** **HTLV-I: human T-cell lymphotrophic virus type I cause of other disease**

HTLV-II B9734

**I10** **HTN: hypertension NOS includes high blood pressure, essential, primary, benign, ma**

SEE hypertension for more htn types/codes
RELATED
history of tobacco dependence Z87891 tobacco use Z720
occupational exposure to environmental tobacco smoke Z5731
Nicotine dependence NOS F17209 SEE Nicotine dependence for more
exposure to environmental tobacco smoke Z7722

**HTR: hemolytic transfusion reaction**

acute d/t Rh incompatibility T80410-
acute d/t ABO incompatibility T80310-
delayed 24 hr+ d/t Rh incompatibility T80411-
delayed 24 hr+ d/t ABO incompatibility T80311-
unspecified d/t Rh incompatibility T80419-
unspecified d/t ABO incompatibility T80319-
7th character indicates encounter
A - initial encounter D - subsequent encounter S - sequela

**E8381** **Hungry bone syndrome**

**G10** **Huntington's chorea**

If dementia present code also one:
without behavioral disturbance F0280
with behavioral disturbance F0281

**D5930** **HUS: hemolytic uremic syndrome unspecified**

Infection-associated D5931
Hereditary D5932 Other D5939
RELATED pneumococcal pneumonia J13
RELATED shigella dyenteriae A039
RELATED e colli infection B962- final character below
NOS 0 STEC 0157 1 other spec STEC 2
other unsp STEC 3 non STEC 9

**N433** **Hydrocele of spermatic cord, testis or tunica vaginalis unspecified**

encysted N430 infected N431 other N432

**G919** **Hydrocephalus NOS**

communicating G910 obstructive G911
normal pressure G912 post trauma NOS G913
in other disease G914 code other disease first
other G918

**N1330** **Hydronephrosis NOS**

w/ureteral stricture NEC N131
w/ renal & ureteral calculous obstruction N132
w/ ureteropelvic junction obstruction N130
other N1339
Pyonephrosis (any above with infection) N136

**N134** **Hydroureter NOS**

nfected N136

**E269** **Hyperaldosteronism NOS (also aldosteronism)**

other primary E2609 Secondary E261
Bartler's E2681 Conn's syndrome E2601
glucocorticoid-remediable E2602

**E7800** **Hyperbetalipoproteinemia**

**E8352** **Hypercalcemia**

**R82994** **Hypercalciuria**

**E7800** **Hypercholesterolemia pure NOS / unspecified**

Familial hypercholesterolemia E7801

**R739** **Hyperglycemia NOS**

post-pancreatectomy E891

**E781** **Hyperglyceridemia endogenous/pure**

mixed E783
w/hypercholesterolemia E782

**E7251** **Hyperglycinemia non-ketotic**

**E875** **Hyperkalemia**

**E785** **Hyperlipidemia unspecified**

Elevated Lipoprotein(a) E7841
Other / Familial combined hyperlipidemia E7849

**E7800** **Hyperlipoproteinemia Fredrickson's type IIa / pure / LDL**

**M4810** **Hyperostosis ankylosing (diffuse idiopathic skeletal) NOS**

occipito-atlanto-axial M4811
cervical M4812 cervicothoracic M4813
thoracic M4814 thoracolumbar M4815
lumbar M4816 lumbosacral M4817
sacral and sacrococcygeal M4818
multiple sites M4819

| | |
|---|---|
| **R82992** | **Hyperoxaluria NOS** |
| | Primary E7253 |
| **E213** | **Hyperparathyroidism NOS** |
| | primary E210 secondary / NEC E211<br>secondary of renal origin N2581<br>other E212 ectopic E342 |
| **D731** | **Hypersplenism** |
| **I10** | **Hypertension essential/primary** |
| | RELATED additional codes if applicable<br>Exposure to environmental tobacco smoke NOS Z7722<br>History of tobacco dependence Z87891<br>Exposure to environmental tobacco smoke occupational Z5731<br>tobacco use Z720<br>Nicotine dependence NOS F17209 SEE Nicotine dependence for more |
| **K766** | **Hypertension portal** |
| | RELATED gastropathy K3189 |
| **I2720** | **Hypertension pulmonary NOS** |
| | Secondary pulmonary arterial hypertension I2721<br>d/t left heart disease I2722<br>d/t lung diseases and hypoxia I2723<br>Chronic thromboembolic I2724<br>Other secondary I2729<br>pulmonary primary I270 |
| **I159** | **Hypertension secondary NOS Code also underlying condition** |
| | renovascular I150 d/t other renal disorders I151<br>d/t endocrine disorders I152 other I158<br>postop I973 DO NOT use this code with any above<br>RELATED<br>exposure to environmental tobacco smoke Z7722<br>history of tobacco dependence Z87891<br>occupational exposure to environmental tobacco smoke Z5731<br>tobacco use Z720 |
| **I169** | **Hypertensive crisis unspecified** |
| | Hypertensive urgency I160<br>Hypertensive emergency I161<br>Code also any identified hypertensive disease<br>RELATED<br>exposure to environmental tobacco smoke Z7722<br>history of tobacco dependence Z87891<br>occupational exposure to environmental tobacco smoke Z5731<br>tobacco use Z720<br>current tobacco dependence SEE nicotine dependence |

**R82993** **Hyperuricoscuria**

**E8351** **Hypocalcemia**

**R82991** **Hypocitraturia**

**E162** **Hypoglycemia NOS**

diabetic: NOS E11649 w/coma E11641
nondiabetic drug induced: NOS E160 w/coma E15
other nondiabetic E161

**E876** **Hypokalemia**

RELATED nephropathy from impaired renal function N2589

**E209** **Hypoparathyroidism NOS**

idiopathic E200 pseudo E201
postop E892 Other E208

**G96810** **Hypotension Intracranial unspecified**

Intracranial hypotension, spontaneous G96811
Intracranial hypotension other G96819
PARTIAL LIST OF RELATED
Brachial amyotrophy G545 Other secondary parkinsonism G218
Cerebrospinal fluid leak from spine G9602
Spinal cord herniation G9589 Syringomyelia G950
Reversible cerebrovascular vasoconstriction syndrome I67841
Nerve root and compressions in diseases classified elsewhere G55

**I959** **Hypotension NOS**

idiopathic I950 d/t drugs I952 Post-procedure NOS I9581
d/t hemodialysis I953 orthostatic/postural I951
chronic/(permanent idiopathic) / other I9589
cardiovascular collapse (shock) R579
nonspecific low blood pressure reading NOS R031
neurogenic orthostatic (Shy-Drager) G903
following ventricular shunting G972

**E039** **Hypothyroidism NOS/primary**

d/t iodine / PAS/ iatrogenic E032
secondary acquired NOS E038
postop or d/t radiation therapy E890
congenital E009 postinfectious E033

**E861** **Hypovolemia - NOT hypovolemic shock, see shock hypovolemic**

Also code associated disorders of electrolyte and acid-base balance below
Hyperosmolality & hypernatremia (Sodium excess) E870
Hypoosmolality & hyponatremia (Sodium deficiency) E871
Acidosis E872 Alkalosis E873
Mixed disorder of acid-base balance E874
Hyperkalemia E875 Hypokalemia E876
Electrolyte imbalance NOS E878

**B0224** **HZM: herpes zoster myelitis**

# I10 Cheat Sheet for Home Care - FY 2023

| | |
|---|---|
| **K5090** | **IBD: inflammatory bowel disease NOS** |
| | SEE Crohn's disease unspecified intestine for more |
| **G7241** | **IBM: inclusion body myositis** |
| **K589** | **IBS: irritable bowel syndrome NOS** |
| | w/ diarrhea K580 w/ constipation K581<br>Mixed K582 Other K588 |
| **N3010** | **IC: interstitial cystitis chronic (also ICC)** |
| | with hematuria N3011 |
| **F79** | **ID: intellectual disability NOS** |
| | mild IQ 50-70 F70 moderate IQ 35-55 F71<br>severe IQ 20-40 F72 profound IQ below 20 F73<br>other F78 |
| **H2181** | **IFIS: intraoperative floppy iris syndrome** |
| **E269** | **IHA: idiopathic hyperaldosteronism** |
| **I259** | **IHD: ischemic heart disease NOS (chronic)** |
| | RELATED history of tobacco dependence Z87891 |
| **I421** | **IHSS: idiopathic hypertrophic subaortic stenosis** |
| **K529** | **Ileitis NOS noninfective** |
| | regional K5000 (Crohn's) |
| **K632** | **Ileorectal fistula** |
| **Z432** | **Ileostomy care / aftercare** |
| | status w/o need for care Z932 |
| **K9410** | **Ileostomy complication NOS** |
| | hemorrhage K9411 malfunction K9413<br>other K9419 infection K9412<br>for infection also code type eg. abd wall cellulitis L03311 or a sepsis<br>granulation of surrounding skin L928 |
| **K560** | **Ileus paralytic/(secondary NOS) of colon or small intestine** |
| | gallstone ileus K563 unspecified ileus K567 |
| **I723** | **Iliac artery aneurysm** |
| **I7772** | **Iliac artery dissection** |

| | | |
|---|---|---|
| **S32309-** | **ilium fracture Unspecified NOS** | |

Unspecified: right ilium S32301- left ilium S32302-
Avulsion Displaced: right S32311- left S32312- unspecified S32313-
Avulsion Nondisplaced: right S32314- left S32315- unspecified S32316-
Other: right S32391- left S32392- unspecified S32399-
Add the appropriate 7th character:
initial encounter: closed fracture= A open fracture= B
subsequent encounter: routine healing= D delayed healing= G
subsequent encounter: routine healing= D delayed healing= G
sequela = S

**Immunization complications**

Infection/Sepsis T880XX-
Rash following immunization T881XX-
postimmunization encephalitis G0402
postimmunization fever R5083
postimmunization arthropathy M022
Add 7th character to T codes:
A - initial encounter D - subsequent encounter S - sequela

**D819** **Immunodeficiency severe combined NOS**

w/ reticular dysgenesis D810
w/ low T and B cell numbers D811
w/ low or normal B cell numbers D812

**D849** **Immunodeficiency unspecified**

Immunodeficiency due to conditions classified elsewhere D8481 Code underlying conditio

Immunodeficiency due to drugs D84821
Immunodeficiency due to external causes D84822
Other immunodeficiencies D8489

**H6120** **Impaction cerumen NOS**

right ear H6121 left ear H6122 bilat H6123

**L0100** **Impetigo NOS**

Non-bullous L0101 Brockhart's/follicularis L0102
Bullous/neonatorum L0103 Other/ulcerative L0109

**E46** **Inanition NOS**

w/edema E43 d/t food deprivation T730XX-
FOR T CODE 7th character indicates encounter
A- initial encounter D- subsequent encounter S- sequela

**K432** **Incisional hernia ventral NOS**

incarcerated K430 gangrenous K431

**G7241** **Inclusion body myositis**

**K30** **Indigestion**

**INFARCTION --SEE Type**

**T880XX-** **Infection following immunization, also sepsis**

7th character indicates encounter
A- initial encounter D- subsequent encounter S- sequela

**INFECTION GENERALIZED -- SEE sepsis, For specific see site, type or source**

**Z1630** **Infection resistant to unspecifed drug**

ampicillin / penicillin Z1611
sulfonamides/ tetracylines / Kanomycin/ Streptomycin Z1629
cephalosporins Z1610 multiple drugs unspec Z1624
quinolones/fluoroquinolones Z1623
Vancomycin Z1621 Vancomycin related Z1622
antivirals Z1633 antifungals Z1632

**T8149x -** **Infection surgical drainage site SEE Postop infection for more**

7th character indicates encounter
A - initial encounter D - subsequent encounter S - sequela

**Infectious agents as the cause of disease - SEE TABLE**

**Influenza & pneumonia RELATED codes**

lung abscess w/pneumonia J851 w/o pneumonia J852
pleural effusion in other conditions J918
sinusitis unsp J0190 unsp recurrent J0191 SEE sinusitis for more
tympanic membrane rupture NOS: unsp ear H7290
tympanic membrane rupture right ear H7291 left ear H7292 bilat H7293

**Influenza d/t identified avian flu virus A/H5N1 (avian / bird / swine)**

w/other respiratory manifestations J09X2
w/gastrointestinal manifestations J09X3
w/other manifestations J09X9

**Influenza d/t novel influenza A virus (avian, bird, swine, H5N1)**

w/pneumonia J09x1
w/other respiratory manifestations J09x2
w/gastrointestinal manifestations J09x3
w/other manifestations J09x9

**Influenza d/t other identified influenza virus**

w/unspecified pneumonia J1000
w/pneumonia d/t same virus J1001
w/pneumonia d/t different virus J1008
w/other respiratory manifestations J101
w/gastrointestinal manifestations J102
w/encephalopathy J1081 w/myocarditis J1082
w/otitis media J1083 w/other manifestations J1089

**J111** **Influenza NOS (d/t unidentified virus)**

w/gastrointestinal manifestations J112
w/encephalopathy J1181 w/myocarditis J1182
w/otitis media J1183 w/other manifestations J1189

| | |
|---|---|
| **Z451** | **Infusion pump adjustment and management** |
| **K4020** | **Inguinal hernia bilateral NOS** |
| | recurrent K4021<br>bilat: w/obstruction NOS K4000 recurrent K4001<br>bilat: w/gangrene NOS K4010 recurrent K4011 |
| **K4090** | **Inguinal hernia unilateral NOS - (right & left code the same)** |
| | recurrent NOS K4091<br>w/ gangrene NOS K4040 recurrent w/gangrene K4041<br>w/obstruction NOS K4030 recurrent w/obstruction K4031 |
| **I889** | **Inguinal lymphadenitis NOS** |
| | acute L041 chronic I881 |
| **G912** | **INPH: idiopathic normal pressure hydrocephalus** |
| | secondary INPH G910 |
| **G4700** | **Insomnia NOS** |
| | d/t medical condition G4701 also code condition<br>primary F5101 d/t mental disorder F5105<br>other NEC G4709 |
| **T383X5-** | **Insulin adverse effect** |
| | 7th character indicates encounter<br>A- initial encounter D- subsequent encounter S- sequela |
| **Z4681** | **Insulin pump fitting & adjustment & training** |
| | Insulin Pump presence Z9641<br>mechanical breakdown T85614-<br>displacement T85624- leakage T85633-<br>infection/inflammation d/t pump T8572x-<br>For T codes, 7th character indicates encounter<br>A- initial encounter D- subsequent encounter S- sequela |
| | **Insulin toxicity** |
| | accidental/NOS T383X1- adverse effect T383X5-<br>underdosing T383X6-<br>7th character indicates encounter<br>A- initial encounter D- subsequent encounter S- sequela |
| **G580** | **Intercostal neuropathy** |

**M51A0** **Intervertebral disc annulus fibrosus defect lumbar unspecified size**

annulus fibrosus defect lumbar small M51A1
annulus fibrosus defect lumbar large M51A2
annulus fibrosus defect lumbosacral unspecified size M51A3
annulus fibrosus defect lumbosacral small M51A4
annulus fibrosus defect lumbosacral large M51A5
IF APPLICABLE code below first -
For A0, A1, A2 above
w/myelopathy M5106 w/radiculopathy M5116
other intervertebral disc displacement M5126
For A4, A5 above
w/ radiculopathy M5117 other intervertebral disc displacement, M5127

**K5650** **Intestinal adhesions postinfection with obstruction NOS**

with partial obstruction K5651
with complete obstruction K5652

**Z4659** **Intestinal appliance fitting & adjustment**

**K56609** **Intestinal obstruction NOS**

Partial unspecified as to cause K56600
Complete unspecified as to cause K56601
Other partial intestinal obstruction K56690
Other complete intestinal obstruction K56691
Other unspecified as to partial vs complete K56699
Postop unspecified as to partial vs complete K9130
Postop partial K9131 Postop complete K9132

**A049** **Intestine infection bacterial NOS**

e. coli Enteropathogenic A040
e. coli Enterotoxigenic A041
e coli Enteroinvasive A042
e coli Enterohemorrhagic A043
e coli other intestinal infection A044
Campylobacter enteritis A045
Yersinia enterocolitica Enteritis A046
Clostridium difficile Enterocolitis A047
Other specified bacterial intestinal infections A048

**C49A4** **Intestine large stromal tumor**

**N8050** **Intestine NOS endometriosis unspecified**

**N80569** **Intestine small NOS endometriosis NOS unspecified depth**

Superficial N80561 Deep N80562

**I69119** **Intracerebral hemorrhage nontraumatic Late effects sequelae cognitive deficits Unsp**

Attention and concentration deficit I69110
Memory deficit I69111 Psychomotor deficit I69113
Visuospatial deficit and spatial neglect I69112
Frontal lobe and executive function deficit I69114
Cognitive social or emotional deficit I69115
Other symptoms and signs involving cognitive functions I69118
Speech and language, fluency disorder I69123

**K614** **Intrasphincteric abscess / cellulitis ( Intersphincteric also)**

**E222** **ISADH: inappropriate secretion of antidiuretic hormone syndrome**

**K6139** **Ischiorectal abscess / cellulitis NOS (also ischioanal)**

Horseshoe abscess K6131

**N3642** **ISD: intrinsic sphincter deficiency (urethral)**

w/ urethral hypermobility N3643

**A073** **Isosporiasis**

**L299** **Itch NOS**

genital unsp L293 vulva L292
perianal L290 ani L290
winter L298 scroti L291
Sarcoptic itch B86

**D693** **ITP: idiopathic thrombocytopenic purpura**

**Z452** **IV catheter adjustment and management**

**T80219-** **IV caused infection unsp infection**

bloodstream infection T80211-
local T80212- other T80218-
7th character indicates encounter
A- initial encounter D- subsequent encounter S- sequela

**M519** **IVDP: interertebral disc prolapse NOS SEE HNP FOR MORE**

**I615** **IVH: intraventricular hemorrhage adult (nontraumatic)**

**Z4803** **Jackson Pratt post op drain change / removal**

**M081** **JAS: juvenile ankylosing spondylitis**

**R17** **Jaundice NOS / symptomatic**

**Joint mice SEE joint site**

**Joint prosthetic complication mechanical unspecified joint**

Change 6th character (9) for specified joint:
0= right hip 1= left hip 2= right knee 3= left knee 8= other
broken T84019- dislocation T84029-
mechanical loosening T84039-
peri prosthetic: fracture T84049- osteolysis T84059-
7th character indicates encounter
A- initial encounter D- subsequent encounter S- sequela

**M0800 JRA: juvenile rheumatoid arthritis NOS**

# I10 Cheat Sheet for Home Care - FY 2023

# K

**C469** **Kaposi's sarcoma NOS**

skin C460 soft tissue C461
palate C462 lymph nodes C463
gastrointestinal sites C464
Lung: unsp C4650 right C4651 left C4652
other sites C467
RELATED: Kaposi's sarcoma associated herpes virus infection B1089

**L821** **Keratosis seborrheic NOS**

inflamed L820
RELATED
Seborrhea capitis L210
Seborrheic infantile dermatitis L211
Other seborrheic dermatitis L218
Seborrheic dermatitis, unspecified L219

**N151** **Kidney abscess/carbuncle/cellulitis**

**N2889** **Kidney adhesions**

**N261** **Kidney atrophy terminal**

**N200** **Kidney calculus**

w/calculus of ureter N202

**N281** **Kidney cyst acquired**

**I129** **Kidney disease chronic hypertensive NOS**

w/stage 5 ckd I120
Also code CKD stage BELOW

**N189** **Kidney disease chronic NOS (CKD)**

stage 1 N181 stage 2 mild N182
stage 3 moderate N183 stage 4 severe N184
stage 5 N185
stage 5 requiring chronic dialysis (ESRD) N186
RELATED dialysis status Z992

**D631** **Kidney disease chronic RELATED anemia**

**N2581** **Kidney disease RELATED hyperparathyroidism secondary**

**N179** **Kidney failure acute NOS**

w/tubular necrosis N170
w/acute cortical necrosis N171
w/medullary necrosis N172
other N178

**N19** **Kidney failure NOS**

**N269** **Kidney fibrosis NOS**

**N2889** **Kidney hemorrhage**

**N2881** **Kidney hypertrophy**

**N280** **Kidney ischemia / infarction**

**N289** **Kidney lesion/mass**

**Kidney neoplasm EXCEPT renal pelvis**

MALIGNANT primary right C641 left C642 unsp C649
Secondary right C7901 left C7902 unsp C7900
Benign right D3001 left D3002 unsp D3000
Mets to bone C7951 mets to unsp lymph nodes C779
Mets to intraabdominal lymph node C772

**Kidney neoplasm RENAL PELVIS**

MALIGNANT primary right C651 left C652 unsp C659
Secondary right C7901 left C7902 unsp C7900
Benign right D3011 left D3012 unsp D3010
Mets to bone C7951 mets to unsp lymph nodes C779
Mets to intraabdominal lymph node C772
Mets to intrapelvic lymph node C775

**N269** **Kidney sclerosis NOS**

**N279** **Kidney small NOS**

unilateral N270 bilateral N271

**N200** **Kidney stone**

w/ureter stone N202

**M4820** **Kissing spine NOS**

occipito-atlanto-axial M4821
cervical M4822 cervicothoracic M4823
thoracic M4824 thoracolumbar M4825
lumbar M4826 lumbosacral M4827

**L03115** **Knee abscess NOS/Right**

left L03116

**M24669** **Knee ankylosis unspecified**

right M24661 left M24662

**Knee arthritis infectious**

in other disease right M01x61 left M01x62 unsp M01x69
pyogenic staph: right M00061 left M00062 unsp M00069
pneumococcal: right M00161 left M00162 unsp M00169
other strep: right M00261 left M00262 unsp M00269
other bacteria: right M00861 left M00862 unsp M00869

**Knee bursitis NOS**

prepatellar: unsp M7040 right M7041 left M7042
other: unsp M7050 right M7051 left M7052

**M71469** **Knee calcification unspecified**

right M71461 left M71462

**M9269** **Knee chondromalacia NOS unspecified**

right M94261 left M94262

**M2240** **Knee chondromalacia patellae NOS unspecified**

right M2241 left M2242

**M24569** **Knee contractures unspecified**

right M24561 left M24562

**M25469** **Knee effusion (joint) unspecified**

right 25461 left M25412

**Knee gout acute/NOS**

idiopathic/primary: right M10061 left M10062 unsp M10069
lead induced: right M10161 left M10162 unsp M10169
drug induced: right M10261 left M10262 unsp M10269
d/t renal impairment: right M10361 left M10362 unsp M10369
other secondary: right M10461 left M10462 unsp M10469

**Knee gout chronic**

idiopathic/primary right M1A061- left M1A062- unsp M1A069-
lead induced right M1A161- left M1A162- unsp M1A169-
drug induced right M1A261- left M1A262- unsp M1A269-
d/t renal impairment right M1A361- left M1A362- unsp M1A369-
other secondary right M1A461- Left M1A462- unsp M1A469-
ADD The appropriate 7th character
0 = without tophus (tophi) 1 = with tophus (tophi)

**M25069** **Knee hemarthrosis unspecified**

right M25061 left M25062

**M2340** **Knee joint mice unspecified**

right M2341 left M2342

**Knee joint prosthetic complication mechanical RIGHT**

Change 6th character for LEFT knee joint = 3
broken T84012- instability T84022-
mechanical loosening T84032-
peri prosthetic: fracture T84042- osteolysis T84052-
wear of articular bearing surface T84062-
7th character indicates encounter
A- initial encounter D- subsequent encounter S- sequela

**M179** **Knee osteoarthritis NOS**

primary: right M1711 left M1712 bilateral M170 unsp M1710
post-trauma: right M1731 left M1732 unsp M1730
other secondary: unilateral M175 bilat M174

**M25569** **Knee pain unspecified**

right M25561 left M25562

**Z96659** **Knee replacement status NOS**

right Z96651 left Z96652 bilat Z96653

**A985** **Korean hemorrhagic fever**

**C469** **KS: Kaposi's sarcoma NOS**

skin C460 soft tissue C461
palate C462 lymph nodes C463
gastrointestinal sites C464
lung: unsp C4650 right C4651 left C4652
other sites C467

**B1089** **KSHVI: Kaposi's sarcoma associated herpes virus infection**

**A982** **Kyasanur Forest disease**

**M40209** **Kyphosis NOS See Tables for more specific**

Code underlying disease first

**M963** **Kyphosis postlaminectomy**

Kyphosis postradiation M962

**Labyrinthine hydrops - SEE Vertigo Meniere's**

R760 **LAC: Lupus anticoagulant finding w/o diagnosis**

Lupus anticoagulant syndrome diagnosis D6862

E739 **Lactose intolerance NOS**

congenital lactase deficiency E730
secondary lactase deficiency E731
other E738

I6381 **Lacunar infarction**

**Lacunar syndromes**

pure motor G465 pure sensory G466 Other G467
Code lacunar infarction I6381 first as etiology for syndromes

G7080 **Lambert-Eaton syndrome NOS**

in neoplastic disease G731 code neoplasm first
in other disease G7081 code underlying disease first

J040 **Laryngitis acute**

acute obstructive J050

J042 **Laryngotracheitis acute**

I69319 **Late effects cerebral infarction sequelae cognitive deficits - Unspecified symptoms an**

Attention and concentration deficit I69310
Memory deficit I69311 Psychomotor deficit I69313
Visuospatial deficit and spatial neglect I69312
Frontal lobe and executive function deficit I69314
Cognitive social or emotional deficit I69315
Other symptoms and signs involving cognitive functions I69318
Speech and language, fluency disorder I69323

I69819 **Late effects cerebrovascular disease OTHER THAN cerebral infarction, subarachnoi**

Attention and concentration deficit I69810
Memory deficit I69811 Psychomotor deficit I69813
Visuospatial deficit and spatial neglect I69812
Frontal lobe and executive function deficit I69814
Cognitive social or emotional deficit I69815
Other symptoms and signs involving cognitive functions I69818
Speech and language, fluency disorder I69823

I69119 **Late effects intracerebral hemorrhage nontraumatic sequelae cognitive deficits Unsp**

Attention and concentration deficit I69110
Memory deficit I69111 Psychomotor deficit I69113
Visuospatial deficit and spatial neglect I69112
Frontal lobe and executive function deficit I69114
Cognitive social or emotional deficit I69115
Other symptoms and signs involving cognitive functions I69118
Speech and language, fluency disorder I69123

**I69019** **Late effects subarachnoid hemorrhage nontraumatic sequelae cognitive deficits Unsp**

Attention and concentration deficit I69010
Memory deficit I69011 Psychomotor deficit I69013
Visuospatial deficit and spatial neglect I69012
Frontal lobe and executive function deficit I69014
Cognitive social or emotional deficit I69015
Other symptoms and signs involving cognitive functions I69018

**I69919** **Late effects unspecified cerebrovascular disease cognitive deficits Unspecified sympto**

Attention and concentration deficit I69910
Memory deficit I69911 Psychomotor deficit I69913
Visuospatial deficit and spatial neglect I698912
Frontal lobe and executive function deficit I69914
Cognitive social or emotional deficit I69915
Other symptoms and signs involving cognitive functions I69918
Speech and language, fluency disorder I69923

**I447** **LBBB: left bundle branch block NOS SEE Heart block for more**

**I4460** **LBBH: left bundle branch hemiblock NOS SEE Heart block for more**

**M5450** **LBP: low back pain NOS**

Vertebrogenic M5451 Other M5459

**M5450** **LBP: low back pain NOS**

Vertebrogenic M5451 Other M5459

**R740** **LDH: lactic acid dehydrogenase elevated blood level**

**L02415** **Leg abscess cutaneous right**

left L02416

**Z899** **Leg amputation status NOS**

above knee: NOS Z89619 right Z89611 left Z89612
at ankle: NOS Z89449 right Z89441 left Z89442
at hip: NOS Z89629 right Z89621 left Z89622
below knee: NOS Z89519 right Z89511 Left Z89512

**I724** **Leg artery aneurysm**

**L02435** **Leg carbuncle right, code organism if known**

left L02436

**G5770** **Leg causalgia unspecified lower limb**

right G5771 left G5772 bilateral G5773

**Leg compartment syndrome - Includes all sites from hip to toes**

nontraumatic: right M79A21 left M79A22 unsp M79A29
traumatic: right T79A21- left T79A22- unsp T79A29-
For traumatic codes, 7th character indicates encounter
A- initial encounter D- subsequent encounter S- sequela

**R252** **Leg cramps NOS**

sleep related G4762 Charley-horse M62831
carpo-pedal spasm R290

**Z86718** **Leg deep vein thrombosis personal history of**

SEE LEG embolism/thrombosis FOR DV THROMBOSIS CODES

**R600** **Leg edema NOS**

**I743** **Leg embolism arterial**

**Leg embolism/thrombosis venous deep ACUTE**

NOS: right I82401 left I82402 bilat I82403 unsp I82409
femoral: right I82411 left I82412 bilat I82413 unsp I82419
iliac: right I82421 left I82422 bilat I82423 unsp I82429
popliteal: right I82431 left I82432 bilat I82433 unsp I82439
tibial: right I82441 left I82442 bilat I82443 unsp I82449

**Leg embolism/thrombosis venous deep CHRONIC**

NOS: right I82501 left I82502 bilat I82503 unsp I82509
femoral: right I82511 left I82512 bilat I82513 unsp I82519
iliac: right I82521 left I82522 bilat I82523 unsp I82529
popliteal: right I82531 left I82532 bilat I82533 unsp I82539
tibial: right I82541 left I82542 bilat I82543 unsp I82549

**Leg fracture pathological NOS / Change 4th character to 5 for 'in neoplastic disease'**

femur unsp M84453- right M84451- left M84452-
tibia right M84461- left M84462-
fibula right M84463- left M84464-
Lower leg unspecified M84469-
7th character indicates encounter/status
A - initial S - sequela
D - subsequent routine healing
G - subsequent delayed healing
K - subsequent nonunion P - subsequent malunion

**L02425** **Leg furuncle/boil right**

left L02426

**G5780** **Leg interdigital neuroma of unspecified lower limb**

right G5781 left G5782 bilateral G5783

**R2240** **Leg lump/mass/swelling skin NOS unspecified lower limb**

right R2241 left R2242 bilat R2243

**G5780** **Leg mononeuropathy other NEC of unspecified lower limb**

right G5781 left G5782 bilateral G5783

**G5790** **Leg mononeuropathy unspecified of unspecified lower limb**

**G8310** **Leg monoplegia NOS**

dominant side: right G8311 left G8312
nondominant: right G8313 left G8314

**Leg osteonecrosis CHOOSE 4th character below**

pelvis: M87-50
femur: unsp M87-59 right M87-51 left M87-52
tibia: unsp M87-63 right M87-61 left M87-62
fibula: unsp M87-66 right M87-64 left M87-65
ankle: unsp M87-73 right M87-71 left M87-72
foot: unsp M87-76 right M87-74 left M87-75
toes: unsp M87-79 right M87-77 left M87-78
ADD 4th character
idiopathic: aseptic = 0 d/t drugs = 1 d/t trauma = 2
other secondary = 3 other = 8

**Leg osteoporosis age related w/current pathological fracture**

femur: unsp M80059- right M80051- left M80052-
lower leg: unsp M80069- right M80061- left M80062-
ankle / foot: unsp M80079- right M80071- left M80072-
7th character indicates encounter/status
A- initial S- sequela D- subsequent routine healing
G- subsequent delayed healing
K- subsequent nonunion P- subsequent malunion

**I743** **Leg peripheral disease occlusive**

**Leg Thrombosis and embolism deep vein specified veins ACUTE**

Acute femoral vein (common/deep) I8241
Acute iliac vein (common/external/internal) I8242
Acute tibial vein (anterior/posterior) I8244
Acute peroneal vein: unspecified I82459
right I82451 left I82452 bilateral I82453
Acute calf muscle vein (gastrocnemial/soleal/NOS): unspecified I82469
right I82461 left I82462 bilateral I82463
FOR CHRONIC change the 4th character (4) to 5

**I8390** **Leg varicose veins NOS or asymptomatic NOS**

asymptomatic: right I8391 left I8392 bilat I8393

**I83899** **Leg varicose veins with other complication unspecified**

other complications: right I83891 left I83892 bilat I83893
with pain: right I83811 left I83812 bilat I83813 unspec I83819

**Leg varicose veins WITH ULCER**

thigh right I83011 left I83021 unspec 83001
calf right I83012 left I83022 unspec 83002
ankle right I83013 left I83023 unspec I83003
heel & midfoot right I83014 left I83024 unspec I83004
other part of foot right I83015 left I83025 unspec I83005
other part lower leg right I83018 left I83028 unspec I83008
unspecified site on leg right I83019 left I83029 unspec I83009
for Leg varicose veins WITH ULCER and INFLAMMATION
Change the 4th character (0) to 2
SEE BELOW for additional code for sevewrity

**Leg varicose veins with ulcer - ADDITIONAL CODES to identify SEVERITY**

skin breakdown: right L97211 left L97221 unsp L97201
fat exposed: right L97212 left L97222 unsp L97202
muscle necrosis: right L97213 left L97223 unsp L97203
bone necrosis: right L97214 left L97224 unsp L97204
unspecified: right L97219 left L97229 unsp L97209

**A481** **Legionnaires' disease**

nonpneumonic Legionnaire's disease A482

**Lemoyez' syndrome SEE vertigo peripheral NOS**

**A279** **Leptospirosis unspecified**

icterohemorrhagica A270 Aseptic meningitis A2781 Other A2789

**C9100** **Leukemia acute lymphoid (ALL) NOS**

in remission C9101 in relapse C9102

**C9200** **Leukemia acute myeloid NOS (AML)**

in remission C9201 in relapse C9202

**C9240** **Leukemia acute promyelocytic NOS (APL)**

in remission C9241 in relapse C9242

**C9110** **Leukemia chronic lymphoid NOS (CLL)**

in remission C9111 in relapse C9112

**C9140** **Leukemia hairy cell NOS**

in remission C9141 in relapse C9142

**I673** **Leukoecephalopathy progressive vascular**

**I456** **LGL: Lown-Ganong-Levine syndrome**

**R87612** **LGSIL: low grade squamous intraepithelial lesion from cervix pap smear**

from vaginal pap smear R87622

**I501** **LHF: left heart failure NOS**

**M3211** **Libman-Sacks disease**

**B852** **Lice NOS**

body B851 head B850
pubic B853 mixed infection B854

**L439** **Lichen planus unspecified**

hypertrophic L430 bullous L431
lichenoid drug rection L432
subacute / tropicus L433 other L438

**R42** **Lightheaded**

**K4090** **LIH: left inguinal hernia NOS -- SEE INGUINAL HERNIA FOR MORE**

**S00531** **Lip bruise / contusion / hematoma**

**E881** **Lipodystrophy NOS (do not use w/Whipple's disease)**

**E882** **Lipomatosis NOS**

**A329** **Listeriosis unspecified**

Cutaneous A320 meningitis A3211
meningoencephalitis A3212 sepsis A327
Oculoglandular A3281 endocarditis A3282
Other A3289

**K750** **Liver abscess NOS**

RELATED
Acute viral hepatitis, unspecified B179
Acute and subacute hepatic failure K7200 w/ coma K7201
Other chronic hepatitis, NEC K738

**K7460** **Liver cirrhosis NOS**

alcoholic: NOS K7030 w/ascites K7031
other/ cryptogenic/ portal/ postnecrotic K7469
pigmentary E83110 w/ toxic liver disease K717
RELATED
esophageal varices I8510 w/bleeding I8511

**K761** **Liver congestion chronic passive**

**Liver disease End stage, Chronic hepatic failure**

chronic: NOS K7210 w/coma K7211

**Liver failure**

acute/ subacute: NOS K7200 w/coma K7201
chronic: NOS K7210 w/coma K7211
unspecified: NOS K7290 w/coma K7291
alcoholic NOS K7040 w/coma K7041

**K760** **Liver fatty NEC**

alcoholic K700

**K7400** **Liver fibrosis unspecified**

early fibrosis stage F1 or stage F2 K7401
advanced fibrosis stage F3 K7402
w/ sclerosis K742
fibrosis & sclerosis alcoholic K702

**K763** **Liver infarction**

**K739** **Liver inflammation NOS**

supperative K750

**K762** **Liver necrosis central hemorrhagic**

IF liver failure is coded, this dx is included

**Liver neoplasms**

MALIGNANT primary
liver cell carcinoma / hepatoma C220
intrahepatic bile duct carcinoma C221
hepatoblastoma C222 primary unsp type C228
angiosarcoma C223 other sarcoma C224
SECONDARY C787 BENIGN D134
not specified primary or secondary / NOS C229
Mets to bone C7951 mets to unsp lymph nodes C779

**K741** **Liver sclerosis**

w/ fibrosis K742

**R55** **LOC: loss of consciousness no trauma NOS (blackout)**

**G835** **Locked-in state**

**J8289** **Löffler's pneumonia**

**I4581** **Long QT syndrome**

**Long term use (current) medications - includes aftercare NEC**

methadone for pain Z79891
antibiotics Z792 aspirin Z7982
anticoagulants Z7901 systemic steroids Z7951
antiplatelet / antithrombotic Z7902
nonsteroidal antiinflammatories Z791

**Lordosis acquired Code underlying disease first**

NOS: unsp M4050 thoracolumbar M4055
NOS: lumbar M4056 lumbosacral M4057
postural: unsp M4040 thoracolumbar M4055
postural: lumbar M4046 lumbosacral M4047
Postop M964

**R630** **Loss of appetite simple NOS**

of nonorganic origin F5089

**M5450** **Low back pain NOS**

Vertebrogenic M5451 Other M5459

**M5450** **Lumbago unspecified**

w/sciatica: unsp M5440 right M5441 left M5442

**Lumbar neuritis or radiculitis SEE Radiculopathy**

**Lumbar puncture complication**

fluid leak G970 headache G971 hemorrhage/hematoma G9751

**J852** **Lung abscess NOS**

w/pneumonia J851

**N80B2** **Lung endometriosis of**

**J850** **Lung gangrene & necrosis**

**Lung neoplasm (and bronchus)**

MALIGNANT primary
bronchus: unsp C3400 right C3401 left C3402
upper lobe bronchus or lung: unsp C3410 right C3411 left C3412
lower lobe bronchus or lung: unsp C3430 right C3431 left C3432
middle lobe C342
overlapping sites bronchus & lung: unsp C3480 right C3481 left C3482
unspecified part bronchus or lung: unsp C3490 right C3491 left C3492
SECONDARY: unsp lung C7800 right C7801 left C7802
BENIGN: unsp D1430 right D1431 left D1432
Mets to bone C7951 mets to unsp lymph nodes C779

**D6862** **Lupus anticoagulant syndrome (LAC)**

LAC finding w/o diagnosis R760

**L930** **Lupus erythematosus non systemic NOS**

subacute cutaneous L931 other L932

**M329** **Lupus erythematosus systemic NOS**

Drug induced M320 w/lung involvement M3213
w/endocarditis M3211 w/pericarditis M3212
w/tubulo-interstitial disease M3215 w/glomerular disease M3214
w/other organ or system involvement M3219
other forms of SLE M328

**LUTS: lower urinary tract symptoms -Code first any cause eg BPH**

Code also any associated overactive bladder N3281
bladder incomplete emptying R3914
nocturia physical R351 psychogenic F458
straining on urination R3916
urinary frequency R350 urinary hesitancy R3911
urinary incontinence NOS R32 see urinary incontinence for more
urinary obstruction N139 urinary retention R339
urinary urgency N3941 weak urinary stream R3912

**A6920** **Lyme disease unspecified**

meningitis A6921 other neurologic disorder A6922
arthritis A6923 other A6929

**Lymph node neoplasms SECONDARY AS METS FROM OTHER NEOPLASMS**

head / face / neck C770 intrathoracic C771
intra-abdominal C772 axilla / arm C773
inguinal / leg C774 intrapelvic C775
multiple regions C778 unsp / NOS C779

**I898** **Lymph node rupture / fistula / infarction**

**I889** **Lymphadenitis NOS**

acute unsp L049 chronic except mesentery I881
mesenteric unsp I880
d/t brugia (wuchereria) malayi B741
d/t wuchereria bancroftia B740
acute: face/neck L040 trunk L041
acute: arm / axilla L042 leg L043

**R591** **Lymphadenopathy NOS same code for generalized enlarged lymph nodes**

localized enlarged nodes R590
enlarged nodes unsp R599

**I891** **Lymphangitis chronic / NOS**

**I890** **Lymphedema acquired/praecox/secondary NOS**

postmastectomy I972

**I898** **Lymphocele any site also chylous ascites, chylous cyst, lymph node rupture**

**C8590** **Lymphoma NOS non-Hodgkin malignant, unspecified site**

SEE TYPE if specified - Burkitt, Hodgkin
head/face/neck C8591 intrathoracic C8592
intra-abdominal C8593 axilla / arm C8594 inguinal / leg C8595
intrapelvic C8596 spleen C8597 multiple C8598 extranodal C8599

# I10 Cheat Sheet for Home Care - FY 2023

A312 **MAC sepsis**

A319 **MAC/MTB: mycobacterium avium complex infection NOS / atypical**

pulmonary A310

**Machine dependence**

respirator Z9911 aspirator Z990
cardiac pacemaker Z950 renal dialysis Z992
supplemental oxygen Z9981
heart assist device Z95811
wheel chair Z993 AICD Z95810

H35329- **Macular degeneration age-related / senile exudative/ wet Unspecified eye**

right eye H35321- left eye H35322- bilateral H35323-
Assign the 7th character from the following
0 - stage unspecified 3 - with inactive scar
1 - with active choroidal neovascularization
2 - with inactive choroidal neovascularization with involuted or regressed neovascularizati

H35319- **Macular degeneration age-related / senile nonexudative/ dry Unspecified eye**

right eye H35311- left eye H35312- bilateral H35313-
Assign the 7th character from the following
0 - stage unspecified 1 - early dry stage
2 - intermediate dry stage
3 - advanced atrophic w/o subfoveal involvement advanced dry stage
4 - advanced atrophic with subfoveal involvement

H3530 **Macular degeneration age-related / senile, NOS/unspecified**

H3530 **Macular degeneration age-related / senile, NOS/unspecified**

H35359 **Macular degeneration cystoid unspecified eye**

right H35351 left H35352 bilateral H35353

H35359 **Macular degeneration cystoid unspecified eye**

right H35351 left H35352 bilateral H35353

H35329- **Macular degeneration exudative (wet) age-related unspecified eye**

right H35321- left H35322- bilateral H35323-
Assign the 7th character from the following
0 - stage unspecified 3 - with inactive scar
1 - with active choroidal neovascularization
2 - with inactive choroidal neovascularization

H35329- **Macular degeneration exudative (wet) age-related unspecified eye**

right H35321- left H35322- bilateral H35323-
Assign the 7th character from the following
0 - stage unspecified 3 - with inactive scar
1 - with active choroidal neovascularization
2 - with inactive choroidal neovascularization

**H35319-** **Macular degeneration nonexudative (dry) age-related unspecified eye**

right H35311- left H35312- bilateral H35313-
Add 7th character to designate the stage
0 - stage unspecified 1 - early dry stage
2 - intermediate dry stage
3 - advanced atrophic without subfoveal involvement
4 - advanced atrophic with subfoveal involvement

**B479** **Madura foot NOS**

mycotic B470

**E8340** **Magnesium metabolism disorder NOS**

hypermagnesemia E8341 hypomagnesemia E8342
other E8349

**K909** **Malabsorption syndrome NOS**

following GI surgery K912
of disaccharides E7439

**E46** **Malnutrition NOS**

kwashiorkor E40 marasmic kwashiorkor E42
nutritional marasmus E41
protein-calorie severe NOS E43 moderate E440 mild E441
retarded development d/t E45

**E710** **Maple syrup urine disease**

**A983** **Marburg virus disease**

**C7952** **Marrow neoplasm SECONDARY / Mets to marrow**

Mets to bone C7951

**D8940** **Mast cell activation disorder/ syndrome, unspecified**

Monoclonal D8941 Idiopathic D8942
Secondary D8943 Code also underlying etiology, if known
Other D8949

**N6120** **Mastitis granulomatous, unspecified breast**

right breast N6121 left breast N6122 bilateral N6123

**N610** **Mastitis if abscess present code breast abscess**

**Mastoiditis acute**

NOS: right H70001 left H70002
bilat H70003 unsp H70009
w/abscess: right H70011 left H70012
right H70011 left H70012
w/other complication: right H70091 left H70092
bilat H70093 unsp H70099

**Mastoiditis CHRONIC**

NOS: unsp H7010 bilat H7013 right H7011 left H7012
unspecified: unsp H7090 bilat H7093 right H7091 Left H7092
in infectious / parasitic disease classified elsewhere -
unsp H7500 bilat H7503 right H7501 left H7502

N6019 **Mastopathy diffuse cystic NOS**

right N6011 left N6012

I671 **MCA: middle cerebral aneurysm**

G3184 **MCI: mild cognitive impairment, so stated Do not use with codes for sequelae of cere**

M303 **MCLS: mucocutaneous lymph node syndrome**

H3530 **MD: macular degeneration NOS (age related) SEE macular degeneration for more**

G7100 **MD: muscular dystrophy NOS except myotonic**

Duchenne or Becker G7101
Facioscapulohumeral G7102
mytonic G7111
Other specified G7109
Limb girdle Autosomal dominant/type 1 G71031
Limb girdle Autosomal recessive/type 2a G71032
Limb girdle muscular dystrophy type 2B G71033
Limb girdle MD due to sarcoglycan dysfunction, unspec G710340
Limb girdle MD due to sarcoglycan dysfunction,alpha G710341
Limb girdle MD due to sarcoglycan dysfunction, beta G710342
Limb girdle MD due to sarcoglycan dysfunction, other G710349
Limb girdle muscular dystrophy type 2L G71035
Limb girdle muscular dystrophy other G71038
Limb girdle muscular dystrophy, unspecified G71039

F339 **MDD: major depressive disorder recurrent episode NOS**

mild F330 moderate F331
severe F332 severe w/psychotic behavior F333
in remission NOS F3340 full remission F3342 partial remission F3341
recurrent brief episodes F338

F329 **MDD: major depressive disorder single episode NOS**

mild F320 moderate F321
severe NOS F322 severe w/psychotic behavior F323
partial or unspecified remission F324
in full remission F325
Depression/Depressive disorder unspecified /NOS F32A

D469 **MDS: myelodysplastic syndrome NOS**

**B059** **Measles NOS**

encephalitis B050 meningitis B051
pneumonia B052 otitis media B053
intestinal complications B054
keratitis and keratoconjunctivitis B0581
Other measles complications B0589

**N342** **Meatitis urethral**

**Medication monitoring SEE Drug level monitoring**

**Medications long term use (current) - includes aftercare SEE Drug Long term use**

**T80219-** **Mediport infection Unspecified (includes Hickman, PIC, portacath, triple lumen etc)**

systemic infection T80211- local infection T80212-
other specified T80218-
7th character indicates encounter
A- initial encounter D- subsequent encounter S- sequela

**K5939** **Megacolon NEC**

Toxic megacolon K5931 identify toxic agent if known / applicable
in Hirschsprung's disease Q431
in Clostridiium difficile recurrent A0471 non-recurrent A0472
in Chaga's disease B5732

**N2882** **Megaloureter**

**C439** **Melanoma malignant unsp / NOS**

lip C430 scalp & neck C434
eyelid: unsp C4310 right C4311 left C431
ear: unsp C4320 right C4321 left C4322
nose C4331 face NOS C4330
other specified parts of face C4339
trunk: anal skin C4351 breast C4352 other C4359
arm/shoulder: unsp C4360 right C4361 left C4362
leg/hip: unsp C4370 right C4371 left C4372
overlapping sites C438
Mets to bone C7951 mets to unsp lymph nodes C779

**R82998** **Melanuria**

**E8841** **MELAS: mitochondrial encephalopathy, lactic acidosis and stroke like episodes**

**K921** **Melena**

**R413** **Memory loss NOS**

**E3120** **MEN: multiple endocrine neoplasia NOS**

type I E3121 type IIA E3122 type IIB E3123
family history Z8341
genetic susceptibility Z1581

**Meninges neoplasm malignant**

cerebral: primary C700 secondary C7932 benign D320
spinal: primary C701 secondary C7949 benign D321
unspecified primary C709 secondary C7949 benign D329

**G01** **Meningitis bacterial in other disease NEC**

RELATED UNDERLYING
leptospirosis A2781 listeriosis A3211
meningococcal A390 neurosyphilis A5213
tuberculosis A170 gonococcal A5481

**G009** **Meningitis bacterial NOS**

nonpyogenic NOS G030 chronic NOS G031
benign recurrent NOS G032
bacterial hemophilus influenzae G000
staphylococcal G003 streptococcal G002
pneumococcal/ d/t Streptococcal pneumoniae G001
bacterial other G008

**G02** **Meningitis nonbacterial in other infectious/parasitic disease**

RELATED UNDERLYING
candida B375 cryptococcal B451 herpes simplex B003
measles meningitis B051 mumps meningitis B261
varicella meningitis B010 rubella meningitis B0602
zoster meningitis B021 coccidioidomycosis B384

**G039** **Meningitis unspecified**

d/t other specified causes G038
USE IF NOT ELSEWHERE LISTED

**A879** **Meningitis viral NOS**

enteroviral A870 adenoviral A871
ymphocytic choriomeningitis A872 other A878

**A399** **Meningococcal infections unspecified**

adrenal syndrome A391 arthritis A3983
postmeningococcal arthritis A3984
carditis unsp A3950 conjunctivitis A3989
encephalitis A3981 endocarditis A3951
meningitis A390 retrobulbar neuritis A3982
meningococcemia: acute A392 chronic A393 unsp A394
myocarditis A3952 pericarditis A3953

**E28319** **Menopause premature asymptomatic**

symptomatic E28310

**G5710** **Meralgia paresthetica unspecified lower limb**

right G5711 left G5712 bilateral G5713

**E8842** **MERRF: myoclonic epilepsy associated with ragged red fibers syndrome**

Code also progressive myoclonic epilepsy from these:
not intractable with status epilepticus G40301
not intractable without status epilepticus G40309
ntractable with status epilepticus G40311
intractable without status epilepticus G40319

**I880** **Mesenteric lymphadenitis acute/chronic/subacute**

**C459** **Mesothelioma unspecified**

pleura C450 pericardium C452
peritoneum C451 includes mesentery, mesocolon, omentum
other sites C457

**R948** **Metabolism basal abnormal**

**Metaplasia gastric intestinal -- SEE gastric intestinal metaplasia**

**I213** **MI: myocardial infarction NOS (any current episode)**

RELATED
exposure to environmental tobacco smoke Z7722
history of tobacco dependence Z87891
occupational exposure to environmental tobacco smoke Z5731
Nicotine dependence NOS F17209 SEE Nicotine dependence for more
tobacco use Z720

**I252** **MI: old myocardial infarction (over 1 year) SEE related at current MI entry**

**M3111** **Microangiopathy thrombotic hematopoietic stem cell transplantation-associated**

Code first if applicable:
Unspecified complication of bone marrow transplant T8600
Bone marrow transplant rejection T8601
Bone marrow transplant failure T8602
Bone marrow transplant infection T8603
Other complications of bone marrow transplant T8609
RELATED:
acute respiratory distress syndrome J80
capillary leak syndrome I788
diffuse alveolar hemorrhage R0489
encephalopathy (metabolic) (septic) G9341
luid overload, unspecified E8770
hemolytic uremic syndrome D593
hepatic veno-occlusive disease K765

**M3119** **Microangiopathy thrombotic other**

**M3110** **Microangiopathy thrombotic unspecified**

**R39198** **Micturition difficulty other**

hesitancy R3911 weak stream R3912
incomplete bladder emptying R3914
urgency R3915 straining R3916
Need to immediately re-void R39191
Position dependent R39192 Extravasation of urine R390

**C717** **Midbrain neoplasm malignant primary**

Secondary C7931 Benign D331

**Mid-foot ulcer non-pressure chronic SEE HEEL**

**G43D0** **Migraine abdominal NOS**

intractable G43D1

**G43709** **Migraine chronic w/o aura NOS**

w/status migrainosus G43701 intractable NOS G43719
intractable w/status migrainosus G43711

**G43009** **Migraine common NOS**

w/status migrainosus G43001 intractable NOS G43019
intractable w/status migrainosus G43011

**G43829** **Migraine menstrual NOS**

w/status migrainosus G43821 intractable NOS G43839
intractable w/status migrainosus G43831

**G43909** **Migraine NOS**

w/status migrainosus G43901 intractable NOS G43919
intractable w/status migrainosus G43911

**G43A0** **Migraine vomiting cyclical**

0

**G43109** **Migraine w/aura, classical NOS**

w/status migrainosus G43101 intractable NOS G43119
intractable w/status migrainosus G43111

**I3481** **Mitral (valve) annulus calcification Nonrheumatic**

Other nonrheumatic mitral valve disorders I3489

**I349** **Mitral valve disorder/disease nonrheumatic NOS**

insufficiency I340 prolapse I341 rheumatic I059
stenosis I342 other I3489
annulus calcification I3481

**G6182** **MMN: Multifocal motor neuropathy**

**B04** **Monkeypox**

**B2790** **MONO: mononucleosis infectious NOS SEE mononucleosis for more**

**G587** **Mononeuritis multiplex**

**G589** **Mononeuropathy unspecified SEE site if known**

**B2790** **Mononucleosis infectious NOS**

mono NOS w/polyneuropathy B2791 w/meningitis B2792
mono NOS w/complication other B2799
Change 4th character if type of virus is specified:
gammaherpesviral = 0 cytomegaloviral = 1
other specified = 8
RELATED hepatitis K77 encephalitis G053

**G8330** **Monoplegia NOS SEE ARM or LEG if specified**

dominant side: right G8331 left G8332
nondominant: right G8333 left G8334

**G1220** **Motor neuron disease, unspecified**

Amyotrophic lateral sclerosis G1221
Progressive bulbar palsy G1222
Primary lateral sclerosis G1223
Familial motor neuron disease G1224
Progressive spinal muscle atrophy G1225
Other motor neuron disease G1229

**I675** **Moyamoya disease**

**A812** **MPL: multifocal progressive leukoencephalopathy**

**E761** **MPS: mucopolysaccharidosis type II**

NOS E763 type I Hurler's E7601
type I Hurler-Scheie E7602 type I Scheie's E760
Morquio A E76210 Morquio B E76211
Morquio unspecifid E76219
Sanfilippo E7622 other specified E7629

**I52** **MPSC: mucopolysaccharidosis cardiopathy Code first mucopolysaccharidosis, "MPS**

**F79** **MR: mental retardation NOS SEE ID for more**

**A4902** **MRSA: methicillin resistant staph aureus infection (not sepsis)**

MRSA as cause of other disease B9562

**A4102** **MRSAS: methicillin resistant staph aureus septicemia / sepsis**

**G35** **MS: multiple sclerosis**

**B9561** **MSSA: methicillin susceptible staph aureus as cause of disease**

**A4101** **MSSAS: methicillin susceptible staph aureus septicemia**

**K1230** **Mucositis oral unspecified**

ulcerative d/t antineoplastic therapy K1231
ulcerative d/t other drugs K1232
ulcerative d/t radiation K1233
other K1239

**C9000** **Multiple myeloma NOS**

n remission C9001 in relapse C9002

**G35** **Multiple sclerosis**

**B269** **Mumps NOS codes below are "mumps with,,,"**

orchitis B260 meningitis B261
encephalitis B262 pancreatitis B263
hepatitis B2681 myocarditis B2682
nephritis B2683 polyneuropathy B2684
arthritis B2685 other complications B2689

**F6810** **Münchausen's syndrome imposed on self / NOS**

predominantly psychological F6811
predominantly physical F6812
combined psychological and physical F6813
imposed on another / Münchausen's by proxy F68A

**M6281** **Muscle weakness generalized**

**G7100** **Muscular dystrophy NOS except myotonic**

Duchenne or Becker G7101
Facioscapulohumeral G7102
Other specified G7109
Mytonic NOS G7111

**J675** **Mushroom worker's lung**

**I349** **MVD: mitral valve disease/disorder NOS**

rheumatic I059 stenosis I342 insufficiency I340
prolapse (MVP) I341 other I3489
regurgitation NOS (MVR) I340
nonrheumatic mitral (valve) annulus calcification I3481

**M7910** **Myalgia unspecified site**

mastication muscle M7911
auxiliary muscles, head and neck M7912
other site M7918
DO NOT code wih fibromyalgia M797 or any Myositis

**G7000** **Myasthenia gravis NOS**

w/acute exacerbation (in crisis) G7001

**B479** **Mycetoma unspecified**

Eumycetoma B470 Actinomycetoma B471

**A319** **Mycobacterial infection unspecified**

Pulmonary A310 Cutaneous A311 Other A318
Disseminated mycobacterium avium-intracellulare complex (DMAC) A312

**C8400** **Mycosis fungoides unspecified site**

head/face/neck C8401 intrathoracic C8402
intra-abdominal C8403 axilla / arm C8404
nguinal / leg C8405 intrapelvic C8406
spleen C8407 multiple C8408 extranodal C8409

**G0482** **Myelitis acute flaccid**

**G0491** **Myelitis NOS**

transverse G373 toxic G92
postinfectious other G054 postimmunization G0402
herpes: zoster B0224 simplex B0082
post chickenpox B0112

**G373** **Myelitis transverse**

**B879** **Myiasis unspecified**

Cutaneous / Creeping B870 Wound / Traumatic B871
Ocular B872 Nasopharyngeal / Laryngeal B873
Aural B874 Genitourinary B8781
Intestinal B8782 other sites B8789

**I515** **Myocardial degeneration**

**I213** **Myocardial infarction acute NOS**

acute subendocardial / non-Q wave (non STEMI) NOS I214
RELATED
exposure to environmental tobacco smoke Z7722
history of tobacco dependence Z87891
occupational exposure to environmental tobacco smoke Z5731
Nicotine dependence NOS F17209 SEE Nicotine dependence for more
tobacco use Z72

**I252** **Myocardial infarction old**

**I510** **Myocardial infarction sequelae cardiac septal defect old**

as current complication following MI:
atrial septal defect I231 ventricular septal defect I232

**I213** **Myocardial infarction ST elevated NOS (STEMI NOS)**

left main coronary artery I2101
left anterior descending coronary artery I2102
other coronary artery of anterior wall I2109
right coronary artery I2111
other coronary artery of inferior wall I2119
left circumflex coronary artery I2121
other sites I2129
RELATED
history of tobacco dependence Z87891
tobacco use Z720
Nicotine dependence NOS F17209 SEE Nicotine dependence for more

**Myocardial infarction SUBSEQUENT within 4 weeks of previous**

STEMI anterior wall I220 STEMI inferior wall I221
NSTEMI NOS I222 STEMI other sites I228
STEMI NOS I229

**I5A** **Myocardial injury non-ischemic / non-traumatic**

Includes acute, chronic, unspecified

**I240** **Myocardial ischemia acute w/MI**

**I401** **Myocarditis acute/subacute giant cell / Fiedler's/ idiopathic/ isolated**

acute NOS I409 NOS / chronic interstitial I514
septic I400 other I408 gonococcal A5483
rheumatic: NOS I090 acute I012

**G253** **Myoclonus**

**G709** **Myoneural disorder unspecified**

**G729** **Myopathy NOS**

inflammatory NOS G7249 critical illness G7281
alcoholic G721 drug induced G720
d/t other toxic agent G722 code agent first
hereditary NOS G719

**E039** **Myxedema NOS**

W/coma E035

# I10 Cheat Sheet for Home Care - FY 2023

**R112** **N&V: nausea and vomiting together NOS**

**K760** **NAFLD: nonalcoholic fatty liver disease**

**Nail disorders**

ingrowing L600 onycholysis L601
onychogryphosis L602 dystrophy L603
Beau's lines L604 yellow nail syndrome L605
other L608 unspecified L609

**E8849** **NARP: neuropathy, ataxia and retinitis pigmentosa syndrome**

**K7581** **NASH: nonalcoholic steatohepatitis**

**C119** **Nasopharynx neoplasm malignant unspecified / NOS**

superior wall C110 posterior wall C111
lateral wall C112 anterior wall C113
overlapping sites C118
SECONDARY C7989 BENIGN D106
METS to lymph node,head, face and neck C770
METS to brain C7931
RELATED
tobacco use Z720
exposure to environmental tobacco smoke Z7722
occupational exposure Z5731
history of tobacco dependence Z8789s1

**R110** **Nausea NOS**

with vomiting R112

**G4452** **NDPH: new daily persistent headache**

**K5530** **NEC: necrotizing enterocolitis unspecified / NOS**

Stage 1 K5531 Stage 2 K5532 Stage 3 K5533

**S144xx** **Neck nerve injury peripheral NEC**

7th character indicates encounter
A- initial encounter D- subsequent encounter S- sequela

**Neoplasm secondary, mets from other site**

abdominal/hepatic/splenic C772 axillary C773
cervical/neck C770 esophageal/diaphragmatic C771
groin/popliteal C774 intrapelvic C775
multiple sites C778 unspecified C779

**N009** **Nephritic syndrome ACUTE NOS CHANGE third character to 1 for 'Rapidly Progr**

w/minor glomerular abnormality N000
w/focal & segmental glomerular lesions N001
w/diffuse membranous glomerulonephritis N002
w/diffuse mesangial proliferative glomerulonephritis N003
w/diffuse endocapillary proliferative glomerulonephritis N004
w/diffuse mesangiocapillary glomerulonephritis N005
w/dense deposit disease N006
w/diffuse crescentic glomerulonephritis N007
w/other morphologic changes N008
with C3 glomerulonephritis N00A

**N039** **Nephritic syndrome CHRONIC NOS**

CHANGE third character to 5 for UNSPECIFIED CHRONIC N. syndrome
w/minor glomerular abnormality N030
w/focal & segmental glomerular lesions N031
w/diffuse membranous glomerulonephritis N032
w/diffuse mesangial proliferative glomerulonephritis N033
w/diffuse endocapillary proliferative glomerulonephritis N034
w/diffuse mesangiocapillary glomerulonephritis N035
w/dense deposit disease N036
w/diffuse crescentic glomerulonephritis N037
w/other morphologic changes N038
w/ C3 glomerulonephritis N03A

**N059** **Nephritis NOS**

w/renal cortical necrosis N171 salt-losing N2889
chronic NOS N039 acute NOS N009

**N200** **Nephrolithiasis NOS**

w/ureter calculus N202

**N289** **Nephropathy NOS**

Toxic NEC N144 analgesic N140
heavy metal N143
d/t other drug N141 d/t unspec drug N142

**N2883** **Nephroptosis**

**Z436** **Nephrostomy care**

**T83512-** **Nephrostomy catheter infected/inflamed - Use additional code to identify infection**

7th character indicates encounter
A- initial encounter D- subsequent encounter S- sequela

**T83092-** **Nephrostomy catheter mechanical complication other**

displacement T83022- leakage T83032-
mechanical breakdown T83012-
7th character indicates encounter
A- initial encounter D- subsequent encounter S- sequela

**N049** **Nephrotic syndrome unspecified**

w/minor glomerular abnormality N040
w/focal & segmental glomerular lesions N041
w/diffuse membranous glomerulonephritis N042
w/diffuse mesangial proliferative glomerulonephritis N043
w/diffuse endocapillary proliferative glomerulonephritis N044
w/diffuse mesangiocapillary glomerulonephritis N045
w/dense deposit disease N046
w/diffuse crescentic glomerulonephritis N047
w/other morphologic changes N048
in amyloidosis/diabetes mellitus/malaria/polyarteritis/systemic lupus N08
w/ C3 glomerulonephritis N04A

**S346xx-** **Nerve injury peripheral abdomen / lower back / pelvis**

7th character indicates encounter
A- initial encounter D- subsequent encounter S- sequela

**G609** **Neuropathy hereditary/idiopathic NOS**

idiopathic progressive G603 hereditary motor & senory G600

**Q8500** **NF: neurofibromatosis unspecified**

NF1 type I Q8501 NF2 type II 8502
Schwannomatosis Q8503 other NF Q8509

**N341** **NGU: non-gonococcal urethritis NOS**

**E119** **NIDDM: non-insulin dependent diabetes mellitus type 2 NOS SEE Diabetes type 2 fo**

**E75249** **Niemann-Pick disease NOS**

type A E75240 type B E75241 type C E75242
type D E75243 other E75248

**E1101** **NKHHC: nonketotic hyperglycemic-hyperosmolar coma in Type 2 diabetes**

**R351** **Nocturia**

**Z91199** **Noncompliance to medical treatment other**

noncompliance with renal dialysis Z9115
Intentional underdosing of medication d/t financial hardship Z91120
Intentional underdosing of medication d/t other reason Z91128
unIntentional underdosing of medication d/t age-related debility Z91130
unIntentional underdosing of medication for other reason Z91138
other noncompliance with medication Z9114
noncompliance w/diet NOS Z91199 d/t finances Z91190 d/t med reason Z91198

**J339** **Nose polyp unspecified**

nasal cavity / choanal J330
polypoid degeneration J331
of sinus J338

**G912** **NPH: normal pressure hydrocephalus**

secondary G910

B9629 **NSTEC: non-shiga toxin producing e coli as cause of disease**

I214 **NSTEMI: non-ST elevation myocardial infarction NOS**

SEE myocardial infarction for more

**Nucleus palposus herniated**

cervical NOS M5030 lumbar M5136 thoracic M5134

H5500 **Nystagmus unspecified**

Congenital H5501 Latent H5502
Visual deprivation H5503
Other forms H5509

# O

| | |
|---|---|
| **M1990** | **OA: osteoarthritis unsp site NOS - SEE site for specific** |
| | primary NOS M1991 post-traumatic NOS M1992<br>secondary NOS M1993 |
| **E669** | **Obese NOS also code BMI if known** |
| | d/t excess calories: NOS E6609 morbid E6601<br>drug induced E661 overweight NOS E663<br>morbid w/alveolar hypoventilation E662<br>other obesity E668 |
| **F09** | **OBS: organic brain syndrome NOS** |
| **F605** | **Obsessive-compulsive personality disorder** |
| | If appropriate may also code the following<br>Mixed obsessional thoughts and acts F422<br>Hoarding disorder F423<br>Excoriation (skin-picking) disorder F424<br>Other OCD F428 |
| **F429** | **OCD: obsessive compulsive disorder unspecified** |
| | Mixed obsessional thoughts and acts F422<br>Hoarding disorder F423<br>Excoriation (skin-picking) disorder F424<br>Other OCD F428<br>If appropriate may also code Obsessive-compulsive personality disorder F605 |
| **K5981** | **Ogilvie syndrome** |
| **E662** | **OHS: obesity hypoventilation syndrome (Pickwickian)** |
| **H6690** | **OM: otitis media NOS include acute / chronic NOS** |
| | right H6691 left H6692 bilateral H6693 |
| **L0882** | **Omphalitis not of newborn** |
| **A981** | **Omsk hemorrhagic fever** |
| **N7092** | **Oophoritis unspecified** |
| | acute N7002 chronic N7012 |
| **G238** | **OPCA: olivopontocerebellar atrophy** |
| | **Orthopedic aftercare** |
| | following joint replacement surgery Z471<br>for removal of internal fixation device Z472<br>following explantation of knee joint prosthesis Z4733<br>following explantation of hip joint prosthesis Z4732<br>following explantation of shoulder joint prosthesis Z4731<br>following scoliosis surgery Z4782<br>following surgical amputation Z4781 also code limb amputated<br>other orthopedic aftercare Z4789 |
| **Z4689** | **Orthopedic brace fitting & adjustment** |

**G4733** **OSA: obstructive sleep apnea (adult or child)**

**M839** **Osteomalacia adult unspecified**

puerperal M830 senile M831
d/t malabsorption M832 d/t malnutrition M833
aluminum bone disease M834
other drug induced M835 other specified M838

**M810** **Osteoporosis NOS (no current fracture) with current fracture SEE site**

age-related/ postmenopausal/ senile M810
drug induced / disuse / postpro / post-trauma M818
localized M816
Personal history of (healed) osteoporosis fracture Z87310

**Z5189** **OT: occupational therapy**

**H60319** **Otitis externa diffuse:unspecified ear**

right H60311 left H60312 bilateral H60313
If specified other infective change 5th character to '9'
If specified swimmers ear change 5th character to '3'
If specified hemorrhagic change 5th character to '2'
candidal B3784
acute noninfective NOS:
right H60501 left H60502 bilateral H60503 unspec H60519

**H65119** **Otitis media acute & subacute allergic NOS unspecified ear**

right H65111 left H65112 bilateral H65113
IF specified recurrent: unspecified ear H65117
right H65114 left H65115 bilateral H65116
RELATED: history of tobacco dependence Z87891

**H65199** **Otitis media acute & subacute mucoid/nonsuppurative unspecified ear**

right H65191 left H65192 bilateral H65193
If specified as recurrent: unspecified ear H65197
right H65194 left H65195 bilateral H65196
RELATED: history of tobacco dependence Z87891

**H6500** **Otitis media ACUTE serous unspecified ear**

right H6501 left H6502 bilateral H6503
If specified recurrent: unspecified ear H6507
right H6504 left H6505 bilateral H6506
RELATED history of tobacco dependence Z87891

**H6520** **Otitis media CHRONIC serous unspecified ear**

right H6521 left H6522 bilateral H6523
CHRONIC mucoid: unspecified ear H6530
right H6531 left H6532 bilateral H6533
CHRONIC allergic: unspecified ear H65419
right H65411 left H65412 bilateral H65413

**H679** **Otitis media in diseases classified elsewhere unspecified ear**

right ear H671 left ear H672 bilat H673

**H6690** **Otitis media NOS UNSP as acute or chronic unspecified side**

right H6691 left H6692 bilateral H6693

**N8340** **Ovary and fallopian tube prolapse and hernia unspecified side**

right N8341 left N83312
IF atrophy of ovary and fallopian tube both:
unspecified N83339 right N83331 left N83332

**N83209** **Ovary cysts unspecified NOS, unspecified side**

NOS right N83201 left N83202
Follicular unsp side N8300 right N8301 left N8302
Corpus luteum unsp side N8310 right N8311 left N8312
Other unsp side N83299 right N83291 left N83292

**N80109** **Ovary endometriosis NOS**

Right unspecified N80101 superficial N80111 deep N80121
Left unspecified N80102 superficial N80112 deep N80122
Bilateral unspecified N80103 superficial N80113 deep N80123
Unspec unspecified N80109 superficial N80119 deep N80129

**Ovary neoplasm**

Malignant primary: unsp C569 right C561 left C562 bilat C563
Secondary: unsp C7960 right C7961 left C7962 bilat C7963
Benign: unsp D279 right D270 left D271
Mets to bone C7951 mets to unsp lymph nodes C779
Mets to intraabdominal lymph node C772
Mets to intrapelvic lymph node C775

**E282** **Ovary polycystic**

**N83519** **Ovary torsion unspecified side (and ovarian pedicle)**

right N83511 left N83512
with fallopian tube N8353

**Overweight - SEE obese**

# I10 Cheat Sheet for Home Care - FY 2023

# P

**I491** **PAC: premature atrial contraction**

**Pacemaker complication**

Embolism T82817- Pain T82847-
Infection and inflammatory reaction T827xx- Use additional code to identify infection
hemorrhage T82837-
7th character indicates encounter
A- initial encounter D- subsequent encounter S- sequela

**Z45018** **Pacemaker fitting & adjustment**

check / test / replace pacemaker battery Z45010

**Z950** **Pacemaker status**

**I498** **Pacemaker wandering**

**I480** **PAF: paroxysmal atrial fibrillation**

PAF: paroxysmal atrial flutter I4892

**T85848-** **Pain d/t prosthetic devices, implants and grafts OTHER**

cardiac T82847- vascular T82848-
genitourinary T8384x- orthopedic T8484x-
nervous system devices T85840-
7th character indicates encounter
A- initial encounter D- subsequent encounter S- sequela

**R52** **Pain NOS SEE also backache, headache, migraine, abdominal and pain syndromes b**

post-thoracotomy: acute G8912 chronic G8922
other postop: acute G8918 chronic G8928
d/t trauma: acute G8911 chronic G8921
neoplasm related G893 Pelvis pain NOS R102 facial R519
Pain on urination NOS R309 dysuria R300

**G890** **Pain syndrome central**

**G894** **Pain syndrome chronic**

This code may be used with codes for specified pain.
This code cannot be used with codes for generalized pain or pain related to psychological f

**Pain syndrome complex regional**

CRPS I:
arm: right G90511 left G90512 bilat G90513 NOS G90519
leg: right G90521 left G90522 bilat G90523 NOS G90529
other site G9059 unsp G9050
CRPS II:
leg: right G5771 left G5772 NOS G5770
arm: right G5641 left G5642 NOS G5640

**C059** **Palate neoplasm malignant primary unspecified**

hard palate C050 uvula C052
soft palate C051 overlapping sites C058
all SECONDARY C7989 all BENIGN D1039
Mets to bone C7951 mets to esophageal nodes C771
Mets to axilla / arm lymph node C773
RELATED: history of tobacco dependence Z87891

**Z515** **Palliative care**

**M300** **PAN: polyarteritis nodosa NOS**

with lung involvement M301 juvenile M302

**Pancreas abscess/(acute necrosis) SEE Pancreatitis acute**

**K862** **Pancreas cyst**

pseudocyst K863

**K869** **Pancreas disease unspecified**

**K8689** **Pancreas disorders other**

atrophy cirrhosis fibrosis Calculus necrosis
non-acute aseptic/fat/NOS necrosis
Same code for all

**K8681** **Pancreas exocrine insufficiency**

**C259** **Pancreas neoplasm malignant primary NOS**

head C250 body C251 overlapping sites C258
tail C252 pancreatic duct C253
endocrine / islets of Langerhans C254
other parts C257
Secondary C7889
Benign: endocrine D137 all other D136
Mets to bone C7951 mets to unsp lymph nodes C779
Mets to abdominal lymph nodes C772
CODE ALSO exocrine pancreatic insufficiency K8681

**K863** **Pancreas pseudocyst**

cyst K862

**K903** **Pancreas steatorrhea**

**K8591** **Pancreatitis acute necrotizing unspecified type NOS**

unspecified type infected K8592
Idiopathic: NOS K8501 infected K8502
Biliary: NOS K8511 infected K8512
Alcohol induced: NOS K8521 infected K8522
Drug induced: NOS K8531 infected K8532
Other: NOS K8581 infected K8582
SEE Pancreatitis acute without for w/o necrosis or infection

**K8590** **Pancreatitis acute without necrosis or infection, unspecified type NOS**

Idiopathic: K8500 Biliary: K8510 Drug induced: K8530
Alcohol induced: K8520 Other: K8580

**K861** **Pancreatitis chronic other -- Code also exocrine pancreatic insufficiency K8681**

alcohol induced chronic K860

**K8689** **Pancreatolithiasis**

**D61818** **Pancytopenia other**

d/t antineoplastic chemotherapy D61810
d/t other drug D61811

**J189** **PAP: primary atypical pneumonia**

**M048** **PAPA: Pyogenic arthritis, pyoderma gangrenosum, and acne syndrome**

**R295** **Paralysis transient**

**G839** **Paralytic syndrome unspecified**

**G8220** **Paraplegia NOS**

complete G8221 incomplete G8222

**Q826** **Parasacral dimple**

**G219** **Parkinsonism secondary unspecified**

malignant neuroleptic syndrome G210
neuroleptic induced G2111 other drug induced G2119
d/t other external agents G212 vascular G214
postencephalitic G213 other secondary G218

**G20** **Parkinson's disease idiopathic/NOS/primary**

dementia w/Parkinsonism G3183
If dementia is present code also one
without behavioral disturbance F0280
with behavioral disturbance F0281

**C07** **Parotid gland neoplasm malignant primary**

secondary C7989 benign D110
Mets to bone C7951 mets to unsp lymph nodes C779
mets to esophageal nodes C771
RELATED: history of tobacco dependence Z87891

**B343** **Parvovirus infection unspecified**

**I471** **PAT: paroxysmal atrial tachycardia**

**Patella disorders**

recurrent dislocate: unsp M2200 right M2201 left M2202
recurrent sublux: unsp M2210 right M2211 left M2212
other derangements: unsp M223x9 right M223x1 left M223x2
chondromalacia: unsp M2240 right M2241 left M2242
other disorder: unsp M228x9 right M228x1 left M228x2
Disorder NOS: unsp M2290 right M2291 left M2292

**Pathological fracture - SEE osteoporosis with pathological fracture at site (Arm, Leg,**

**Patient education**

diabetes/ diet/ obesity Z713
exercise / injury prevention Z7189
insulin pump Z4681
medications / treatment plan Z7189
tobacco abuse counseling Z716

**R3982** **PBS: painful bladder syndrome**

**E282** **PCOS: polycystic ovary syndrome**

**B59** **PCP: pneumonia/pneumocytosis d/t pneumocystis carinii/jiroveci**

**D45** **PCV: polycythemia vera**

**R600** **Pedal edema**

**PEDICULOSIS - SEE lice**

**N80389** **Pelvic brim endometriosis NOS**

Superficial - right N80361 left N80362 bilateral N80363 unspec N80369
Deep - right N80371 left N80372 bilateral N80373 unspec N80379
Unspecified - right N80381 left N80382 bilateral N80383 unspec N80389

**N803C9** **Pelvic endometriosis uterosacral ligament NOS**

Superficial - right N803A1 left N803A2 bilateral N803A3 unspec N803A9
Deep - right N803B1 left N803B2 bilateral N803B3 unspec N803B9
Unspecified - right N803C1 left N803C2 bilateral N803C3 unspec N803C9

**N80D9** **Pelvic nerves endometriosis other**

Unspecified / NOS N80D0
sacral splanchnic nerves N80D1
sacral nerve roots N80D2
obturator nerve N80D3
sciatic nerve N80D4
pudendal nerve N80D5
femoral nerve N80D6

**N8030** **Pelvic peritoneum endometriosis NOS**

Anterior cul-de-sac - superficial N80311 deep N80312 unspecified N80319
Posterior cul-de-sac - superficial N80321 deep N80322 unspecified N80329

**N80399** **Pelvic peritoneum endometriosis other specified sites unspecified depth**

other specified sites superficial N80391
other specified sites deep N80392

**N80359** **Pelvic sidewall endometriosis NOS**

Superficial - right N80331 left N80332 bilateral N80333 unspec N80339
Deep - right N80341 left N80342 bilateral N80343 unspec N80349
Unspecified - right N80351 left N80352 bilateral N80353 unspec N80359

**N733** **Pelvis abscess female acute**

chronic N734 NOS N735

**Pelvis abscess MALE SEE Peritonitis**

**N736** **Pelvis adhesions female postinfective**

postop N994 (male / female)

**Pelvis bone cyst**

solitary cyst: unsp M85459 right M85451 left M85452
aneurysmal cyst: change 4th character to 5
other cyst: change 4th character to 6

**N9489** **Pelvis congestion syndrome**

**M84454-** **Pelvis fracture pathological**

Change 4th character to 5 for 'in neoplastic disease'
7th character indicates encounter/status
A - initial S - sequela
D - subsequent routine healing
G - subsequent delayed healing
K - subsequent nonunion P - subsequent malunion

**N8182** **Pelvis fundus incompetence/weakening**

**N739** **Pelvis inflammatory disease NOS female**

chronic N731 acute N730
in other disease N74
CODES FOR SOME POSSIBLE UNDERLYING diseases:
tuberculous A1817 chlamydia trachomatis A5611
syphilitic (secondary) A5276 trichomoniasis A5909
gonococcal pelvic inflammatory disease A5424
herpes simplex pelvic inflammatory disease A6009

**N8184** **Pelvis muscle wasting female**

**R102** **Pelvis pain NOS**

**S346xx-** **Pelvis peripheral nerve injury**

7th character indicates encounter
A- initial encounter D- subsequent encounter S- sequela

**R1900** **Pelvis swelling, mass, lump NOS**

Generalized R1907 Other R1909

**I862** **Pelvis varices**

**L109** **Pemphigus NOS**

vulgaris L100 vegetans L101 foliaceous L102
Brazilian L103 erythematosus L104 drug induced L105
paraneoplastic L1081 other L1089

**B484** **Penicillosis**

**E7489** **Pentosuria essential**

**K279** **Peptic ulcer NOS used with no site given or gastroduodenal**

acute: w/hemorrhage K270 w/perforation K271
acute: NOS K273 w/both hemorrhage/perforation K272
chronic/unsp: w/hemorrhage K274 w/perforation K275
chronic/unsp w/both hemorrhage/perforation K276
chronic NOS K277

**K610** **Perianal abscess / cellulitis**

**I309** **Pericardial effusion acute NOS I309**

Pericardial effusion malignant noninflammatory I3131
Other pericardial effusion noninflammatory I3139

**I319** **Pericarditis NOS**

acute nonspecific idiopathic I300 acute infective I301
acute unsp I309 other acute I308
chronic adhesive I310 chronic constrictive I311
gonococcal A5483 coxsackie (virus) B3323
meningococcal A3953 syphilitic A5206
rheumatoid (arthritis) M0531 tuberculosis A1884
in systemic lupus erythematosus M3212
in other disease I32 Code first underlying disease

**Perichondritis ear external**

right: NOS H61001 acute H61011 chronic H61021
left: NOS H61002 acute H61012 chronic H61022
bilat: NOS H61003 acute H61013 chronic H61023
unsp: NOS H61009 acute H61019 chronic H61029

**R102** **Perineal pain NOS**

**N8181** **Perineocele**

**L02215** **Perineum abscess cutaneous**

abscess deep w/urethral involvement N340

**L02225** **Perineum boil / furuncle**

**L02235** **Perineum carbuncle**

**B356** **Perineum infection fungal**

**G96191** **Perineural cyst**

**R579** **Peripheral circulation failure**

**R600** **Peripheral insufficiency venous NOS**

**I739** **Peripheral vascular disease NOS**

**N736** **Peritoneal pelvic adhesions postinfective / NOS female**

postop N994

**Peritoneum & retroperitoneum neoplasm**

MALIGNANT primary
retroperitoneum C480 peritoneum unsp / NOS C482
specified parts of peritoneum C481
overlapping sites of peritoneum & retroperitoneum C488
SECONDARY both the same C786
BENIGN Retroperitoneum D200 Peritoneum D201
Mets to bone C7951 mets to unsp lymph nodes C779
Mets to intraabdominal lymph node C772

**K659** **Peritonitis NOS / acute NOS / bacterial NOS**

chronic proliferative or d/t urine K658
d/t bile K653 spontaneous bacterial K652
generalized: acute K650 w/acute appendicitis K352
gonococcal A5485 Chlamydial A7481
female pelvic NOS N735

**R1033** **Periumbilical pain**

**N340** **Periurethral abscess**

**G5730** **Peroneal nerve palsy unspecified lower limb**

right G5731 left G5732 bilateral G5733

**R233** **Petechiae**

**M048** **PFAPA: Periodic fever, aphthous stomatitis, pharyngitis & adenopathy syndrome**

**G547** **Phantom limb syndrome NOS**

w/ pain G546

**J029** **Pharyngitis acute NOS**

chronic J312 streptococcal J020
w/ unsp flu NOS J111 Gonococcal A545

**G3101** **Pick's disease**

RELATED dementia NOS F0280
RELATED dementia w/behavioral disturbance F0281

**E662** **Pickwickian syndrome**

**PID: Pelvic inflammatory disease female SEE PELVIS inflammatory disease**

**PID: prolapsed intervertebral disc w/myelopathy**

thoracic M5104 lumbar M5106
thoracolumbar M5105

**J8289** **PIE: pulmonary infiltration w/eosinophilia**

**Pilonidal cyst and sinus**

cyst: NOS L0591 w/abscess L0501
sinus/fistula: NOS L0592 w/abscess L0502
sacral dimple congenital or Parasacral dimple Q826

**D075** **PIN: prostate intraepithelial neoplasia type III**

type I or II or NOS (histologically confirmed) N4231
Code types l - ll with type lll if applicable

**B80** **Pinworm**

RELATED vaginitis / vulvitis N771

**E236** **Pituitary abscess**

**E230** **Pituitary cachexia / insufficiency NOS**

postprocedure E893 drug induced E231

**E229** **Pituitary hyperfunction NOS**

**B361** **Pityriasis nigra**

L42 Pityriasis rosea B360 Pityriasis versicolor

**D5521** **PK: (or PKA) pyruvate kinase deficiency anemia**

**E700** **PKU: phenylketonuria**

**A209** **Plague unspecified**

Bubonic A200 Cellulocutaneous A201
Pneumonic A202 meningitis A203
Septicemic A207
Other / Abortive / Asymptomatic A208

**G5760** **Plantar nerve lesion NOS**

right G5761 left G5762 bilateral G5763

**B070** **Plantar warts**

**E8802** **Plasminogen deficiency Type 1 / Type 2**

RELATED
hydrocephalus G914 l igneous conjunctivitis H1051
respiratory disorder related to plasminogen deficiency J99
Otitis media in diseases classified elsewhere:
right ear H671 left ear H672 bilateral H673 unspecified H679

**N80B1** **Pleura endometriosis**

**F3281** **PMDD: premenstrual dysphoric / tension disorder**

**A812** **PML: progressive multifocal leukoencephalopathy**

**M353** **PMR: polymyalgia rheumatica**

with giant cell arteritis M315

**N943** **PMS: premenstrual syndrome (tension)**

RELATED Migraines
not intractable: NOS G43829 w/status migrainosus G43821
intractable: NOS G43839 w/status migrainosus G43831

**R0600** **PND: paroxysmal nocturnal dyspnea NOS**

**J64** **Pneumoconiosis unspecified**

coalworker's J60 asbestosis J61
talc dust J620 silica other than talc J628
aluminosis J630 bauxite fibrosis J631
berylliosis J632 graphite fibrosis J633
siderosis J634 stannosis J635
d/t other inorganic dust J636 in tuberculosis J65

**B59** **Pneumocystosis**

**J159** **Pneumonia bacterial NOS/If concurrent w/influenza, code flu first**

Chlamydial J160 d/t Escherichia coli J155
d/t Klebsiella pneumoniae J150 d/t Pseudomonas J151
d/t Mycoplasma pneumoniae J157
d/t staphylococcus NOS J1520
d/t staph aureus NOS J15211
d/t staph aureus methicillin resistant J15212
d/t other staph J1529
d/t strep pneumoniae J13
d/t streptococcus, group B J153
d/t other streptococci J154

**J8282** **Pneumonia eosinophilic acute**

**J8281** **Pneumonia eosinophilic chronic**

**J849** **Pneumonia interstitial NOS - first code cause if known**

idiopathic NOS J84111 desquamative J84117
lymphoid J842 endogenous lipoid J8489

**J8289** **Pneumonia Löffler's**

**J189** **Pneumonia unspecified organism NOS/If concurrent w/flu, code flu first**

Bronchopneumonia NOS J180 Lobar J181
hypostatic J182 other type unspecified organism J188

**J129** **Pneumonia viral NOS If concurrent w/influenza, code flu first**

adenoviral J120 respiratory synctial virus J121
parainfluenza J122 Human metapneumovirus J123
SARS-associated coronavirus J1281
other viral J1289

**T148xx-** **PNI: peripheral nerve injury NOS**

abdomen / lower back / pelvis S346xx-
neck S144xx-
7th character indicates encounter
A- initial encounter D- subsequent encounter S- sequela

**M300** **Polyarteritis nodosa NOS**

with lung involvement M301 juvenile M302

**M301** **Polyarteritis with lung involvement**

**D45** **Polycythemia vera**

**R631** **Polydipsia**

**M3320** **Polymyositis, organ involvement unspecified**

with respiratory involvement M3321
with myopathy M3322
With other organ involvement M3329

**G63** **Polyneuropathy in other diseases NEC**

Code underlying disease first
Do not use this code for polyneuropathy in:
diabetes, diphtheria, MONO, Lyme disease, mumps,
postherpetic, rheumatoid arthritis, scleroderma, SLE

**G629** **Polyneuropathy NOS**

inflammatory NOS G619 serum G611
drug induced G620 alcoholic G621
radiation induced G6282 critical ilkness G6281
d/t other toxic agent G622
Multifocal motor neuropathy G6182
chronic inflammatory demyelinating G6181
acute postinfective G610 other G6189
in SLE M3219 in Lyme disease A6922
postherpetic B0223 in mumps B2684

**Polyneuropathy sequelae - code first the resulting condition**

to Guillain-Barre' syndrome G650
to other inflammatory polyneuropathy G651
to toxic polyneuropathy G652

**R632** **Polyphagia**

**R3589** **Polyuria NOS**

Nocturnal polyuria R3581
frequency of micturition R350 nocturia R351
psychogenic polyuria F458
RELATED enlarged prostate N401

**E7402** **Pompe disease**

G5730 **Popliteal lateral nerve lesion unspecified lower limb**

right G5731 left G5732 bilateral G5733

G5740 **Popliteal medial nerve lesion unspecified lower limb**

right G5741 left G5742 bilateral G5743

E8020 **Porphyria NOS**

acute intermittent (hepatic) E8021
hereditary erythropoietic E800
cutanea tarda E801
other E8029

I970 **Postcardiotomy syndrome**

G8383 **Posterior cord syndrome**

K911 **Postgastrectomy syndrome**

I237 **Postinfarction angina**

M963 **Postlaminectomy kyphosis**

M961 **Postlaminectomy syndrome**

F070 **Postleucotomy syndrome - Code first underlying physiological condition**

I972 **Postmastectomy lymphedema syndrome**

N951 **Postmenopausal climacteric symptoms**

Includes flushing, sleeplessness, lack of concentration, headache

N959 **Postmenopausal disorder NOS**

bleeding / hemorrhage N950 atrophic vaginitis N952
climacteric states N951 other N958

I241 **Postmyocardial infarction syndrome**

T800XX- **Postop air embolism from infusion / transfusion / injection**

7th character indicates encounter
A- initial encounter D- subsequent encounter S- sequela

J95812 **Postop air leak**

H5940 **Postop bleb inflammation/infection NOS (eye)**

stage 1 H5941 stage 2 H5942 stage 3 H5943

K912 **Postop blind loop syndrome**

Z483 **Postop care cancer/neoplasm - Also code neoplasm**

**Postop Care SEE Aftercare also**

T8189X- **Postop complication NOS**

7th character indicates encounter
A- initial encounter D- subsequent encounter S- sequela

Z4803 **Postop drainage change or removal**

R5082 **Postop fever**

**T8183X-** **Postop fistula persistent**

7th character indicates encounter
A- initial encounter D- subsequent encounter S- sequela

**K911** **Postop gastric surgery syndrome**

**Postop hematoma / hemorrhage DIGESTIVE system**

following digestive system procedure K91840
following other procedure K91841

**Postop hematoma / hemorrhage EAR & MASTOID PROCESS**

following procedure on the ear and mastoid process H9541
following other procedure H9542

**Postop hematoma / hemorrhage ENDOCRINE system**

following an endocrine system procedure E89810
following other procedure E89811

**Postop hematoma / hemorrhage GENITOURINARY system**

following a genitourinary procedure N99820
following other procedure N99821

**Postop hematoma / hemorrhage MUSCULOSKELETAL system**

following a musculoskeletal procedure M96830
following other procedure M96831

**Postop hematoma / hemorrhage OPHTHALMIC system (eye & adnexa)**

following an ophthalmic procedure:
right H59311 left H59312 bilat H59313 unsp H59319
following other procedure:
right H59321 left H59322 bilat H59323 unsp H59329

**Postop hematoma / hemorrhage RESPIRATORY system**

following respiratory system procedure J95830
following other procedure J95831

**Postop hematoma / hemorrhage SKIN & SUBCUT system**

following a dermatologic procedure L7621
following other procedure L7622

**Postop hematoma NERVOUS system**

following a nervous system procedure G9761
following other procedure G9762

**Postop hematoma/hemorrhage CIRCULATORY system**

following cardiac catheterization I97610
following cardiac bypass I97611
following other circulatory system procedure I97618
following other procedure I9762

**Postop hemorrhage NERVOUS system**

following a nervous system procedure G9751
following other procedure G9752

| | |
|---|---|
| **K432** | **Postop hernia ventral NOS** |
| | w/gangrene K431 incarcerated K430 |
| **E891** | **Postop hyperglycemia / hypoinsulinemia** |
| **E892** | **Postop hypoparathyrodism** |
| **E893** | **Postop hypopituitarism** |
| **I9581** | **Postop hypotension (not d/t hemodialysis)** |
| **E890** | **Postop hypothyroidism** |
| | **Postop infarct (cerebrovascular)** |
| | following cardiac surgery I97820<br>following other surgery I97821 |
| **T8140X-** | **Postop infection NOS any site, any except OB** |
| | superficial incisional surgical site T8141X-<br>deep incisional surgical site T8142X-<br>organ and space surgical site T8143X-<br>other surgical site (eg drainage) T8149X-<br>Sepsis following a procedure T8144X-<br>7th character indicates encounter<br>A- initial encounter D- subsequent encounter S- sequela |
| **M6140** | **Postop muscle calcification or ossification unsp site** |
| **K912** | **Postop nonabsorption NOS** |
| **E8940** | **Postop ovary failure asymptomatic** |
| | symptomatic E8941 |
| | **Postop pain** |
| | acute other than thoracotomy G8918<br>acute/NOS postthoracotomy G8912<br>chronic other than postthoracotomy G8928<br>chronic postthoracotomy G8922 |
| **J95811** | **Postop pneumothorax** |
| **M960** | **Postop pseudoarthrosis after fusion or arthrodesis any site** |
| | arthrodesis status Z981 |
| **K6811** | **Postop retroperitoneal abscess -Also code Postop infection if applicable** |
| **T8110X-** | **Postop shock NOS** |
| | cardiogenic T8111X-<br>septic T8112X- Code first underlying infection<br>other/ hypovolemic T8119X-<br>7th character indicates encounter<br>A- initial encounter D- subsequent encounter S- sequela |
| **E895** | **Postop testicle hypofunction** |
| **K910** | **Postop vomiting after gastrointestinal surgery** |

| | |
|---|---|
| | **Postop wound aftercare SEE wound care** |
| **F0781** | **Posttraumatic brain syndrome non-psychotic** |
| **F4310** | **Posttraumatic stress disorder NOS** |
| | acute F4311 chronic F4312 |
| **G90A** | **POTS: Postural orthostatic tachycardia syndrome** |
| **B960** | **PPLO: pleuropneumonia-like organism infection cause of other disease** |
| | pleuropneumonia-like organism pneumonia J157 |
| **R7303** | **Prediabetes** |
| **I6783** | **PRES: posterior reversible encephalopathy syndrome** |
| | **Pressure ulcer - SEE site** |
| **N4832** | **Priapism** |
| **I639** | **PRIND: prolonged resolving or reversible ischemic neurologic deficit** |
| | personal history Z8673 |
| **A819** | **Prion disease of the central nervous system NOS** |
| | If dementia present code also one:<br>without behavioral disturbance F0280<br>with behavioral disturbance F0281 |
| **K627** | **Proctitis d/t radiation** |
| | RELATED radiation therapy Y842 |
| **K6289** | **Proctitis NOS** |
| **K5100** | **Proctitis ulcerative chronic unspecified** |
| | w/rectal bleeding K51011<br>w/intestinal obstruction K51012<br>w/fistula K51013 w/abscess K51014<br>w/other specified complication K51018<br>w/unspecified complication K51019 |
| **K5229** | **Proctocolitis Allergic / Food-induced** |
| **G7111** | **PROMM: proximal myotonic myopathy** |
| **N412** | **Prostate abscess** |
| **N4289** | **Prostate atrophy** |
| **N420** | **Prostate calculus / stone** |
| **N421** | **Prostate congestion and hemorrhage** |
| **N4283** | **Prostate cyst** |
| **N429** | **Prostate disorder NOS** |

**N4230** **Prostate dysplasia unspecified**

Prostatic intraepithelial neoplasia PIN I, PIN II N4231
intraepithelial neoplasia III (PIN III) D075
Atypical small acinar proliferation N4232
Other dysplasia of prostate N4239

**N400** **Prostate enlarged NOS**

WITH lower urinary tract symptoms (LUTS) N401
Also code applicable LUTS below
bladder incomplete emptying R3914
nocturia physical R351 psychogenic F458
straining on urination R3916
frequency R350 hesitancy R3911
urinary obstruction N139 retention R339
urgency N3941 weak urinary stream R3912
urinary incontinence NOS R32 see urinary incontinence for more

**N4289** **Prostate fistula/infarction**

**N421** **Prostate hemorrhage**

**N400** **Prostate hyperplasia/ hypertrophy benign /NOS**

w/LUTS N401 also code LUTS (see @ PROSTATE ENLARGED)

**Prostate intraepithelial neoplasia**

type I or II or NOS (histologically confirmed) N423
type III D075

**C61** **Prostate neoplasm malignant primary**

secondary C7982 benign D291
Mets to bladder C7911 Mets to bone C7951
Mets to unsp lymph nodes C779
Mets to intraabdominal lymph node C772
Mets to intrapelvic lymph node C775
Mets to lymph node,inguinal and lower limb C774
RELATED
Hormone resistant malignancy status Z192
Hormone sensitive malignancy status Z191
Rising PSA following tx for malignant prostate neoplasm R9721

**N402** **Prostate nodular NOS**

w/LUTS N403 also code LUTS (see @ PROSTATE ENLARGED)

**N4281** **Prostate painful syndrome (prostadynia syndrome)**

**R9720** **Prostate specific antigen abnormal**

Rising PSA following tx for prostate malignancy R9721

**N420** **Prostate stone**

**N4289** **Prostate stricture**

**I868** **Prostate varices**

**N419** **Prostatitis NOS**

acute N410 chronic N411
granulomatous N414 other N418
trichomonal A5902 in actinomycosis N51
gonococcal: acute A5422 chronic A5422

**N413** **Prostatocystitis**

**N4282** **Prostatosis syndrome**

**A079** **Protozoal intestinal disease unspecified**

**Z1611** **PRSA: penicillin resistant staph aureus infection (first code infection) - do not use wit**

Code may be used to identify any penicillin resistant infection

**L299** **Pruritis NOS**

genital unsp L293 perianal / ani L290
senilis L298 scroti L291 vulva L292

**R9720** **PSA: prostate specific antigen elevated**

Rising PSA following tx for prostate malignancy R9721

**K8301** **PSC: primary sclerosing cholangitis**

**M960** **Pseudoarthrosis d/t fusion or arthrodesis**

**G932** **Pseudotumor**

**K6812** **Psoas muscle abscess**

**L22** **Psoriasiform napkin eruption /erythema /diaper rash**

**L409** **Psoriasis NOS**

vulgaris L400 generalized pustular L401
guttate L404 pustulosis L403
arthropathic unsp L4050
distal interphalangeal arthropathy L4051
arthritis mutilans L4052 other arthropathic L4059
spondylitis L4053 juvenile arthropathy L4054
other psoriasis L408

**M340** **PSS: progressive systemic sclerosis**

**I471** **PSVT: Paroxysmal supraventricular tachycardia**

**D681** **PTA: plasma thromboplastin antecedent deficiency**

**D67** **PTC: plasma thromboplastin component deficiency**

**D47Z1** **PTLD: post-transplant lymphoproliferative disorder**

**D6951** **PTP: post-transfusion purpura**

**F4310** **PTSD: post traumatic stress disorder NOS**

acute F4311 chronic F4312

**R791** **PTT: partial thromboplastin time abnormal**

| | | |
|---|---|---|
| **K279** | **PUD: peptic ulcer disease NOS -- SEE PEPTIC ULCER FOR MORE** |
| **J984** | **Pulmolithiasis NOS** |
| **J8402** | **Pulmonary alveolar microlithiasis** |
| | alveolar proteinosis J8401 |
| **I281** | **Pulmonary artery aneurysm NOS** |
| **I288** | **Pulmonary artery arteritis/endarteritis/rupture/stenosis/stricture** |
| **J810** | **Pulmonary edema acute** |
| | chronic / NOS J811 |
| **I2699** | **Pulmonary embolism NOS** |
| | septic w/acute cor pulmonale I2601<br>w/saddle embolus of pulmonary artery w/cor pulmonale I2602<br>other w/cor pulmonale I2609<br>septic NOS I2690 (code underlying infection first)<br>saddle embolism NOS I2692<br>chronic I2782<br>RELATED<br>personal hx of pulmonary embolism Z86711<br>long term use of anticoagulants Z7901 |
| **J8410** | **Pulmonary fibrosis unspecified** |
| **I2720** | **Pulmonary hypertension NOS** |
| | pulmonary primary I270<br>Secondary pulmonary arterial hypertension I2721<br>due to left heart disease I2722<br>due to lung diseases and hypoxia I2723<br>Chronic thromboembolic pulmonary hypertension I2724<br>Other secondary pulmonary hypertensio I2729 |
| **R918** | **Pulmonary infiltrate NOS found on imaging** |
| **I379** | **Pulmonary valve disorder nonrheumatic unspecified** |
| | stenosis I370 insufficiency I371<br>stenosis w/insufficiency I372 other I378 |
| **D692** | **Purpura NOS/nonthrombocytopenic NOS/senile** |
| | allergic/ anaphylactoid D690<br>primary annularis telaniectodes L959<br>posttransfusion D6951<br>hypergammaglobulinemic D890<br>fibrinolytic/fulminans D65 |
| **I493** | **PVC: premature ventricular contractions** |
| **I739** | **PVD: peripheral vascular disease NOS** |

**I4720** **PVT: paroxysmal ventricular tachycardia unspecified**

Torsades de pointes I4721 (Code also, if applicable, long QT syndrome I4581)
Other ventricular tachycardia I4729

**Q8711** **PWS: Prader-Willi syndrome**

**N2884** **Pyelitis cystica**

**N12** **Pyelonephritis NOS (also pyelitis)**

acute N10 chronic NOS N119
chronic nonobstructive reflux associated N110
chronic obstructive N111
chronic nonobstructive NOS N118
calculous NOS N209 in other diseases N16

**N2885** **Pyeloureteritis cystica**

**K311** **Pyloric obstruction/stenosis acquired**

**K313** **Pylorospasm NEC**

**K2960** **Pylorus erosion**

w/hemorrhage K2961

**L080** **Pyoderma NOS any site**

gangrenous L88 vegetans L0881

**R8281** **Pyuria**

**G8250** **Quadriplegia NOS**
complete C1-C4 G8251
complete C5-C7 G8253
incomplete C1-C4 G8252
incomplete C5-C7 G8254

**M069** **RA: rheumatoid arthritis (except spine or juvenile) NOS**

**G5630** **Radial nerve lesion unspecified upper limb**
right G5631 left G5632 bilateral G5633

**Z5189** **Radiation therapy convalescence**
Radiation RELATED cystitis N3040 w/hematuria N3041

**M5410** **Radiculopathy unspecified**
occipito-atlanto-axial M5411
cervical M5412 cervicothoracic M5413
thoracic M5414 thoracolumbar M5415
umbar M5416 lumbosacral M5417
sacral and sacrococcygeal M5418

**D4620** **RAEB: refractory anemia with excess blasts NOS**
RAEB-1: refractory anemia with excess blasts-1 D4621
RAEB-2: refractory anemia with excess blasts-2 D4622

**D461** **RARS: refractory anemia with ring sideroblasts**

**R21** **Rash NOS**
diaper L22 heat L740
drug induced: generalized L270 localized L271
food induced L272

**M0500** **RASK: rheumatoid arthritis with splenomegaly and leukopenia NOS aka Felty's syn**

**A259** **Rat bite fevers NOS**
spirillosis (Sodokui) A250 streptobacillosis A251

**I7300** **Raynaud's syndrome NOS**
w/gangrene I7301

**I4510** **RBBB: right bundle branch block NOS**
other I4519 Right fascicular block I450

**D46A** **RCMD: refractory cytopenia with multilineage dysplasia**
w/ ring sideroblasts (RCMD RS) D46B

**J80** **RDS: respiratory distress syndrome acute NOS**

**K611** **Rectal abscess / cellulitis**

**K604** **Rectal fistula**

**N816** **Rectocele female**
male K623

**Rectum disorders**

cyst NOS K6289 endometriosis N805
fissure K602 fistula K603
gonorrhea A546 hemorrhage K625
granuloma/ irritation NOS K6289
infection d/T chlamydia trachomatis A563
polyp NOS K621 polyp adenomatous D128
prolapse except hemorrhoids K623
skin tags K644
stenosis/stricture K624
stromal tumor C49A5
ulcer NOS/ solitary/ stercoral K626

**N80519** **Rectum endometriosis NOS unspecified depth**

Superficial N80511 Deep N80512

**C20** **Rectum Neoplasm malignant primary**

secondary C785 benign D128
Mets to bone C7951 mets to unsp lymph nodes C779
Mets to intraabdominal lymph node C772
Mets to intrapelvic lymph node C775

**Renal artery disorders**

Renal artery aneurysm I722
Renal artery atherosclerosis I701
Renal artery dissection I7773

**N289** **Renal insufficiency acute**

chronic N189

**N269** **Renal sclerosis NOS**

**Z1620** **Resistance to antibiotics NOS**

Resistance to antibiotics - beta lactam type NOS Z1610
Extended spectrum beta lactamase Z1612
penicillins Z1611 beta lactam other Z1619
vancomycin Z1621 vancomycin related Z1622
quinolones / fluoroquinilones Z1623
multiple Z1624 other Z1629

**Z9911** **Respirator dependence**

**J398** **Respiratory disease upper tract NOS**

**J80** **Respiratory distress acute**

**Respiratory failure**

acute: NOS J9600 w/hypoxia J9601 w/hypercapnia J9602
chronic: NOS J9610 w/hypoxia J9611 w/hypercapnia J9612
unsp: NOS J9690 w/hypoxia J9691 w/hypercapnis J9692
Acute w/chronic: NOS J9620 w/hypoxia J9621 w/hypercapnia J9622
postop acute J95821 postop acute with chronic J95822

**M3130** **Respiratory granulomatosis necrotizing NOS**

w/renal involvement M3131

**J393** **Respiratory hypersensitivity reaction NOS**

**J069** **Respiratory infection upper acute NOS (URI)(code infectious agent if known)**

**Respiratory pain**

on respiration R071 precordial pain R072
pleurodynia R0781 intercostal pain R0782
anterior chest wall pain R0789

**G2581** **Restless legs syndrome**

**H3560** **Retina hemorrhage unspecified**

bilateral H3563 right H3561 left H3562

**K6811** **Retroperitoneal abscess postprocedural**

**G937** **Reyes syndrome**

RELATED
adverse effect of aspirin T39015-
adverse effect of other salicylates T39095-
If not an adverse effect, list T39 code before syndrome and change 6th character:
1=accidental 2=intended self harm 3=assault 4=undetermined
7th character below indicates encounter
A- initial encounter D- subsequent encounter S- sequela

**D569** **RGM: Rietti-Greppi-Micheli anemia**

**I099** **RHD: rheumatic heart disease NOS**

**J309** **Rhinitis allergic NOS**

d/t pollen J301 other seasonal J302
d/t food J305 d/t animal hair J3081
other J3089 vasomotor J300

**J310** **Rhinitis chronic**

RELATED CODES
tobacco use Z720 history of tobacco use Z87891
Nicotine dependence NOS F17200
exposure to environmental tobacco smoke Z7722
occupational exposure to environmental tobacco smoke Z5731

**Rib fracture**

One rib: right S2231x- left S2232x- unspecified S2239x
Multiple: right S2241x- left S2242x- bilat S2243x- unspec S2249x
Add the appropriate 7th character:
A - initial encounter for closed fracture
B - initial encounter for open fracture
D - subsequent encounter for closed fracture with routine healing
G - subsequent encounter for closed fracture with delayed healing
K - subsequent encounter for closed fracture with nonunion
S - sequela

**E550** **Rickets active, d/t vitamin D deficiency**

**K4090** **RIH: right inguinal hernia SEE INGUINAL HERNIA FOR MORE**

**I639** **RIND: reversible ischemic neurological deficit**

RIND-hx personal history Z8673

**B359** **Ringworm NOS**

Scalp / Beard B350 nails B351
Hand B352 Foot B353
body B354 Groin B356

**H35179** **RLF: retrolental fibroplasia NOS**

right H35171 left H35172 bilateral H35173

**G2581** **RLS: restless legs syndrome**

**L719** **Rosacea unspecified**

Perioral dermatitis L710
Rhinophyma L711 Other rosacea L718

**Rotator cuff syndrome (nontraumatic)**

complete: unsp M75120 right M75121 left M75122
incomplete: unsp M75110 right M75111 Left M75112
unspecified: unsp M75100 right M75101 left M75102

**B779** **Roundworm unspecified**

w/intestinal complications B770
w/pneumonia B7781
w/other complication B7789

**B974** **RSV: respiratory synctial virus infection as cause of other disease**

Do Not use with the following:
respiratory synctial virus pneumonia J121
acute bronchitis due to respiratory syncytial virus J205
acute bronchiolitis due to respiratory syncytial virus J210

**B069** **Rubella NOS**

w/ neurological complication unsp B0600
encephalitis B0601 meningitis B0602
w/other neuro complications B0609
pneumonia B0681 arthritis B0682
other complications B0689

**I823** **RVT: renal vein thrombosis**

# I10 Cheat Sheet for Home Care - FY 2023

# S

**Q826** **Sacral dimple congenital**

**S332XX-** **Sacroiliac dislocation**

7th character indicates encounter
A= initial encounter D=subsequent S=sequela

**S336XX-** **Sacroiliac sprain**

7th character indicates encounter
A= initial encounter D=subsequen t S=sequela

**M461** **Sacroiliitis NOS**

**S3219x-** **Sacrum fracture Other**

Sacrum fracture Unspecified S3210x-
Sacrum fractures Transverse:
Type 1 flexion fracture with posterior displacement S3214x-
Type 2 flexion fracture with posterior displacement S3215x-
Type 3 extension fracture with anterior displacement S3216x-
Type 4 segmental comminution of upper sacrum S3217x-
Add the appropriate 7th character for sacrum fractures:
initial encounter: closed fracture =A open fracture =B
subsequent encounter: routine healing =D delayed healing =G
subsequent encounter fracture w/nonunion =K
sequela =S

**Sacrum fractures Vertical**

Nondisplaced: Zone I S32110- Zone II S32120- Zone III S32130-
Minimally displaced: Zone I S32111- Zone II S32121- Zone III S32131-
Severely displaced: Zone I S32112- Zone II S32122- Zone III S32132-
Unspecified: Zone I S32119- Zone II S32129- Zone III S32139-
Add the appropriate 7th character:
initial encounter: closed fracture =A open fracture =B
subsequent encounter: routine healing =D delayed healing =G
subsequent encounter fracture w/ nonunion =K
sequela =S

**L89159** **Sacrum ulcer pressure NOS**

unstageable L89150 stage 1 L89151
stage 2 L89152 stage 3 L89153 stage 4 L89154
pressure induced deep tissue damage L89156

**A029** **Salmonella infection NOS**

localized NOS A0220 meningitis A0221
pneumonia A0222 arthritis A0223
osteomyelitis A0224 pyelonephritis A0225
sepsis A021 enteritis A020
other localized infection A0229
other specified A028

**N7091** **Salpingitis unspecified**

Chronic N7011 Acute N7001 gonococcal A5429

**N8340** **Salpingocele unspecified side**

right N8341 left N8342

**D869** **Sarcoidosis NOS**

lung D860 lymph nodes D861
lung & lymph nodes D862 skin D863
meningitis D8681 myocarditis D8685
multiple cranial nerve palsies D8682
pyelonephritis D8684 arthropathy D8686
myositis D8687 other sites D8689

**B86** **Sarcoptic itch**

**B9721** **SARS-severe acute respiratory syndrome, coronavirus infection**

Above code is used for "as cause of other disease"
pneumonia J1281 acute URI J069
exposure to Z2089
observation for suspected exposure Z2001
coronavirus infection unsp B342

**I339** **SBE: subacute bacterial endocarditis**

infective I330

**K56609** **SBO: small bowel obstruction NOS**

Partial unspecified as to cause K56600
Complete unspecified as to cause K56601
Other partial intestinal obstruction K56690
Other complete intestinal obstruction K56691
Other unspecified as to partial vs complete K56699
Postop unspecified as to partial vs complete K9130
Postop partial K9131 Postop complete K9132

**K912** **SBS: short bowel syndrome**

**F458** **SBS: shy bladder syndrome**

**B86** **Scabies**

**I2542** **SCAD: spontaneous coronary artery dissection**

RELATED history of tobacco dependence Z87891

**A389** **Scarlet fever NOS**

with otitis media A380
with myocarditis A381
with other complications A388
RELATED streptococcal sore throat J020

**D571** **SCD: sickle-cell disease NOS**

w/unsp crisis D5700 & thalassemia D57419
w/acute chest syndrome D5701 & thalassemia D57411
w/ splenic sequestration D5702 & thalassemia D57412
sickle-cell thalassemia NOS D5740
with cerebral vascular involvement D5703
with crisis with other specified complication D5709

**Z8241** **SCD: sudden cardiac death family history**

**F209** **Schizophrenia NOS**

paranoid F200 disorganized F201
catatonic F202 residual F205
undifferentiated / atypical F203
schizophreniform psychosis F2081
cyclic F250 other F2089

**G5700** **Sciatic nerve lesion NOS**

right G5701 left G5702 bilateral G5703
Do not use with Sciatica

**M5430** **Sciatica unspecified**

right M5431 left M5432
w/lumbago: unsp M5440 right M5441 left M5442

**D819** **SCID: severe combined immunodeficiency NOS**

w/reticular dysgenesis D810
w/low T and B cell numbers D811
w/low or normal B cell numbers D812

**M419** **Scoliosis NOS any level**

d/t radiation NOS M965 thoracogenic NOS M4130
idiopathic infantile NOS M4100 idiopathic NOS M4120

**N5082** **Scrotum pain**

**E54** **Scurvy**

**L219** **Seborrhea NOS**

Seborrhea capitis L210
Seborrheic infantile dermatitis L211
Other seborrheic dermatitis L218

**A419** **Sepsis / septicemia NOS**

**A4150** **Sepsis d/t gram negative organisms NOS**

d/t E. coli A4151 d/t Pseudomonas A4152
d/t Serratia A4153 other gram negative sepsis A4159

**A413** **Sepsis d/t Hemophilus influenzae**

**A4101** **Sepsis d/t staph aureus NOS**

Methicillin resistant A4102 (MRSA)

**A412** **Sepsis d/t staph NOS**

**A409** **Sepsis d/t strep unspecified**

group A A400 group B A401
s. pneumoniae A403 other A408
Use after cause code, like, postop strep sepsis T814xx-
for T code, 7th character indicates encounter
A- initial encounter D- subsequent encounter S- sequela

**B007** **Sepsis Herpesviral - aka Disseminated herpesviral disease**

**T8144x-** **Sepsis postprocedure NOS also code organism if known**

post immunization T880xx- postop strep sepsis T814xx-
local d/t IV T80212- bloodstream d/t IV T80211-
other d/t IV T80218- unspecified d/t IV T80219-
7th character indicates encounter
A- initial encounter D- subsequent encounter S- sequela
RELATED if applicable Severe sepsis R6520

**R6520** **Sepsis severe NOS**

RELATED
acute kidney failure N179 SEE kidney failure for more
critical illness: myopathy G7281 polyneuropathy G6281
disseminated intravascular coagulopathy D65
septic encephalopathy G9341
sepsis NOS A419 bloodstream infection d/t IV T80211-
postop infection SEE Sepsis postprocedure above (code first)
For T code, 7th character indicates encounter
A - initial encounter D - subsequent encounter S - sequela

**Sequelae - SEE late effects or source condition**

**C8410** **Sezary disease unspecified site**

head/face/neck C8411 intrathoracic C8412
intra-abdominal C8413 axilla/arm C8414
inguinal/leg C8415 intrapelvic C8416
spleen C8417 multiple C8418 extranodal C8419

**A039** **Shigellosis unspecified / bacillary dysentery NOS**

d/t Shigella dysenteriae / group A A030
d/t Shigella flexneri / group B A031
d/t Shigella boydii / group C A032
d/t Shigella sonnei / group D A033
d/t other A038

**B029** **Shingles NOS for specified complications see herpes zoster**

**T782XX-** **Shock anaphylactic NOS**

reaction to food unsp T7800x- d/t peanuts T7801x-
d/t shellfish T7802x- d/t eggs T7808x-
d/t other fish T7803x- d/t milk and dairy T7807x-
d/t blood / blood products T8051x-
d/t vaccination T8052x- d/t other serum T8059x-
adverse effect of medicine T886xx-
7th character indicates encounter
A- initial encounter D- subsequent encounter S- sequela

**R571** **Shock hypovolemic NOS**

postprocedural T8119x-
traumatic T794xx-
For post-op & traumatic 7th character indicates encounter
A- initial encounter D- subsequent encounter S- sequela

**R579** **Shock NOS**

cardiogenic R570
hypovolemic NOS R571
other R578

**Shock postop SEE Postop shock**

**K912** **Short bowel syndrome**

**M24619** **Shoulder ankylosis NOS**

right M24611 left M24612

**Shoulder bone cyst**

solitary: unsp M85419 right M85411 left M85412
aneurysmal: unsp M85519 right M85511 left M85512
other cyst: unsp M85619 right M85611 left M85612

**M7550** **Shoulder bursitis unspecified**

right M7551 left M7552

**M7500** **Shoulder capsulitis adhesive unspecified**

right M7501 left M7502

**M94219** **Shoulder chondromalacia unspecified**

right M94211 left M94212

**M24519** **Shoulder contractures unspecified**

right M24511 left M24512

**M24319** **Shoulder dislocation pathological NOS unspecified**

right M24311 left M24312

**M24419** **Shoulder dislocation recurrent unspecified**

right M24411 left M24412

**M25419** **Shoulder effusion (joint) unspecified**

right M25411 left M25412

**Shoulder fracture pathological NOS / Change 4th character to 5 for 'in neoplastic dis**

unsp M84419- right M84411- left M84412-
7th character indicates encounter/status
A - initial S - sequela
D - subsequent routine healing
G - subsequent delayed healing
K - subsequent nonunion P - subsequent malunion

**Shoulder gout chronic**

idiopathic/primary right M1A011- left M1A012- unsp M1A019-
lead induced right M1A111- left M1A112- unsp M1A119-
drug induced right M1A211- left M1A212- unsp M1A219-
d/t renal impairment right M1A311- left M1A312- unsp M1A319-
other secondary right M1A411- left M1A412- unsp M1A419-
Add appropriate 7th character
0= without tophus (tophi) 1= with tophus (tophi)

**M25019** **Shoulder hemarthrosis unspecified**

right M25011 left M25012

**M7540** **Shoulder impingement syndrome unspecified**

right M7541 left M7542

**M24819** **Shoulder joint instability NOS unspecified**

right M24811 left M24812

**M24019** **Shoulder joint mice unspecified**

right M24011 left M24012

**M19019** **Shoulder osteoarthritis primary unspecified**

right M19011 left M19012

**M80019-** **Shoulder osteoporosis age related w/current fracture unspecified**

right M80011- left M80012-
7th character indicates encounter/status
A - initial D - subsequent routine healing
G - subsequent delayed healing S - sequela
K - subsequent nonunion P - subsequent malunion

**M25519** **Shoulder pain (joint) unspecified**

right M25511 left M25512

**Shoulder rotator cuff syndrome (rotator cuff rupture) non-traumatic**

NOS: unsp M75100 right M75101 left M75102
incomplete: unsp M75110 right M75111 left M75112
complete: unsp M75120 right M75121 left M75122

**M25619** **Shoulder stiffness of joint NOS unspecified**

right M25611 left M25612

**M7530** **Shoulder tendinitis calcifying unspecified**

right M7531 left M7532

**G2583** **Shuddering benign attacks**

**D571** **Sickle-cell disease NOS**

w/unsp crisis D5700 & thalassemia D57419
w/acute chest syndrome D5701 & thalassemia D57411
w/ splenic sequestration D5702 & thalassemia D57412
sickle-cell thalassemia NOS D5740

**D643** **Sideroblastic anemia NOS**

Hereditary sideroblastic anemia D640
Secondary d/t disease D641 Code first underlying disease
Secondary d/t drugs and toxins D642 Code first poisoning due to drug or toxin
Use additional code for adverse effect, if applicable, to identify drug

**N80529** **Sigmoid colon endometriosis NOS unspecified depth**

Superficial N80521 Deep N80522

**Sinusitis ACUTE**

NOS: unspecified J0190 unspecified recurrent J0191
maxillary: unsp J0100 recurrent J0101
frontal: unsp J0110 recurrent J0111
ethmoidal: unsp J0120 recurrent J0121
sphenoidal: unsp J0130 recurrent J0131
pansinusitus: unsp J0140 recurrent J0141
other: unsp J0180 recurrent J0181

**J329** **Sinusitis CHRONIC NOS**

maxillary J320 frontal J321 ethmoidal J322
sphenoidal J323 pansinusitis J324 other J328

**SIRS common underlying infections, code before SIRS**

dt venous cath: local T80212- bloodstream T80211-
other T80218- NOS T80219- d/t procedure T814xx-
d/t transfusion/infusion/injection: blood products T8022x- other T8029x-
For T codes above, 7th character indicates encounter
For T codes above, 7th character indicates encounter
d/t gram negative NOS A4150 d/t enterrococcus A4181
d/t MSSA A4101 d/t MRSA A4102 d/t serratia A4153
d/t unsp staph A412 d/t hemophilus influenzae A413
sepsis: NOS A419 d/t e coli A4151 d/t pseudomonas A4152

**SIRS organ dysfunction common RELATED codes**

acute respiratory failure NOS J9600 w/hypoxia J9601 w/hypercapnia J9602
myopathy G7281 polyneuropathy G6281
acute kidney failure: NOS N179 w/tubular necrosis N170
w/cortical necrosis N171 w/medullary necrosis N172
encephalopathy G9341 DIC D65

**R6510** **SIRS: systemic inflammatory response syndrome non-infectious NOS**

noninfectious w/ acute organ dysfunction R6511
INFECTIOUS R6520 w/septic shock R6521
Use additional code to identify specific acute organ dysfunction
SEE SIRS related codes and infections above

**M7540** **SIS: subacromial impingement syndrome NOS unsp side**

right M7541 left M7542

**L513** **SJS-TEN: Stevens-Johnson syndrome toxic epidermal necrolysis overlap syndrome**

just SJS is coded L511

**R239** **Skin changes NOS**

desquamation/induration/scaling R234
petechiae R233 clammy R231

**L729** **Skin cyst follicular unspecified**

epidermal L720 pilar L7211 sebaceous L723
trichodermal L7212 other L728

**R229** **Skin lump/mass/swelling NOS**

head R220 neck R221 trunk R222
Arm: NOS R2230 right R2231 left R2232 bilat R2233
Leg: NOS R2240 right R2241 left R2242 bilat R2243

**L98499** **Skin ulcer chronic non-pressure other NOS, (back/buttocks separate codes)**

breakdown of skin L98491
fat layer exposed L98492
necrosis of muscle L98493
necrosis of bone L98494
muscle involvement without necrosis L98495
bone involvement without necrosis L98496
other specified severity L98498

**S43439-** **SLAP: superior glenoid labrum lesions NOS**

right S43431- left S43432-
7th character indicates encounter
A- initial encounter D- subsequent encounter S- sequela

**M329** **SLE: Lupus erythematosus systemic NOS**

Drug induced M320 w/lung involvement M3213
w/endocarditis M3211 w/pericarditis M3212
w/tubulo-interstitial disease M3215
w/glomerular disease M3214
w/other organ or system involvement M3219
other forms of SLE M328

**G4730** **Sleep apnea NOS code first any underlying condition**

primary central / idiopathic G4731
obstructive / apnea hypopnea G4733
in other conditions G4737
other specified G4739

**G3182** **SNE: subacute necrotizing encephalopathy**

**R0602** **SOB: short of breath**

**R900** **SOL: space occupying lesion intracranial**

**J029** **Sore throat NOS acute**

chronic J312

**A389** **Sore throat Streptococcal**

RELATED Use a scarlet fever code if applicable
Scarlet fever NOS A389
Scarlet fever with otitis media A380
Scarlet fever with myocarditis A381
Scarlet fever with other complications A388

**G5139** **Spasm clonic hemifacial unspecified**

right G5131 left G5132 bilateral G5133

**N433** **Spermatic cord hydrocelle unspecified**

encysted N430 infected N431 other N432

**Spinal puncture complication**

cerebrospinal fluid leak G970 headache G971
hemorrhage/hematoma G9751

**M4800** **Spine stenosis / caudal stenosis unspecified**

occipito-atlanto-axial M4801
cervical M4802 cervicothoracic M4803
thoracic M4804 thoracolumbar M4805
lumbar NOS M48061 lumbosacral M4807
lumbar with neurogenic claudication M48062
sacral and sacrococcygeal M4808

**D7881** **Spleen complication intraoperative other**

hemorrhage/hematoma complicating procedure on the spleen D7801
hemorrhage/hematoma complicating other procedure D7802
puncture & laceration during procedure on the spleen D7811
Accidental puncture & laceration during other procedure D7812

**D7889** **Spleen complication postop other**

hemorrhage following procedure on the spleen D7821
hemorrhage following other procedure D7822
hematoma following procedure on the spleen D7831
hematoma following other procedure D7832
seroma following a procedure on the spleen D7833
seroma following other procedure D7834

**Spleen disorders**

atrophy D730 hypersplenism D731
chronic congestive splenomegaly D732
abscess D733 cyst D734
infarction / rupture / torsion D735
neutropenic splenomegaly D7381
fibrosis / splenitis NOS D7389
unspecified D739 splenomegaly NOS R161
fibrosarcoma C261

**R948** **Spleen function test abnormal NOS**

**Spleen neoplasm**

malignant primary C261
secondary C7889 benign D139
Mets to bone C7951 mets to unsp lymph nodes C779
Mets to intraabdominal lymph node C772

**R161** **Splenomegaly NOS**

neutropenic D7381 chronic congestive D732

**A0819** **SRV:small round virus NOS infection of intestine (enteritis,gastroenteropathy)**

**E8582** **SSA: Senile systemic amyloidosis**

**A811** **SSPE: subacute sclerosing panencephalitis**

**I495** **SSS: sick sinus syndrome**

**L00** **SSS: staphylococcal scalded skin syndrome (also SSSS)**

**B958** **Staphylococcus infection NOS as cause of disease**

specified other than aureus B957
SEE INFECTIOUS TABLE FOR MORE

**K7581** **Steatohepatitis nonalcoholic**

**B9623** **STEC: shiga toxin producing e coli NOS**

STEC 0157 B9621 other STEC B9622

**I213** **STEMI: ST elevation myocardial infarction NOS**

SEE myocardial infarction ST elevated for more
RELATED
exposure to environmental tobacco smoke Z7722
history of tobacco dependence Z87891
occupational exposure to environmental tobacco smoke Z5731
Nicotine dependence NOS F17209 SEE Nicotine dependence for more
tobacco use Z720

**G2582** **Stiff-man syndrome**

**R413** **STM: short term memory (loss)**

**Stoma infection SEE type, eg colostomy, tracheostomy**

**K31819** **Stomach and duodenum angiodysplasia**

w/bleeding K31811

**K3189** **Stomach congestion passive**

**K3182** **Stomach dieulafoy lesion hemorrhagic**

**K310** **Stomach dilatation/distention acute**

**Stomach neoplasm**

MALIGNANT Primary
body C162 cardia C160 pyloric antrum C163
pylorus C164 lesser curvature C165 unspecified C169
greater curvature C166 fundus C161
overlapping sites C168
Malignant SECONDARY all sites C7889
BENIGN all sites D131
Mets to bone C7951 mets to unsp lymph nodes C779
Mets to intraabdominal lymph node C772

**K312** **Stomach stenosis/stricture hourglass type non congenital**

**C49A2** **Stomach stromal tumor**

**STOMACH ULCER -- SEE gastric**

**K289** **Stomal ulcer unsp NOS**

acute: NOS K283 w/hemorrhage K280 w/perforation K281
acute: w/both hemorrhage & perforation K282
chronic / unsp: NOS K287 w/hemorrhage K284
chronic / unsp: w/perforation: K285
chronic / unsp: w/both hemorrhage & perforation K286

**A690** **Stomatitis acute necrotizing ulcerative (Vincent's)(gangrenous)**

Necrotizing ulcerative (acute) gingivostomatitis A691

**B0861** **Stomatitis bovine**

epizootic B088 herpetic B002

**R195** **Stool abnormality bulky/ color/ fat/ mucus/ occult blood/ pus**

**K921** **Stools black (melana) - do not use w/ulcer**

**J020** **Strep throat pharyngitis**

**B955** **Streptococcus infection NOS as cause of disease**

group A B950 group B B951
group C B954 group G B954
group D (enterococcus) B952
s. pneumoniae B953

**I639** **Stroke NOS SEE Cerebral infarction for more**

**Stroke score, National Institutes of Health Stroke Scale (NIHSS)**

Code first the cerebral infarction (I63-)
NIHSS score 0 R29700 NIHSS score 1 R29701
NIHSS score 2 R29702 NIHSS score 3 R29703
Scores range from 0 to 42 using pattern above
R297xx where xx equals the score

**R401** **Stupor (semi-coma)**

**I69123** **Stuttering as late effect intracerebral hemorrhage nontraumatic**

**I69019** **Subarachnoid hemorrhage nontraumatic sequelae cognitivedeficits Unspecified symp**

Attention and concentration deficit I69010
Memory deficit I69011
Visuospatial deficit and spatial neglect I69012
Psychomotor deficit I69013
Frontal lobe and executive function deficit I69014
Cognitive social or emotional deficit I69015
Other symptoms and signs involving cognitive functions I69018

**I69039** **Subarachnoid hemorrhage nontraumatic sequelae Monoplegia ARM unspecified -- C**

-- tO Code for leg: change 5th character to 4
right dominant side I69031
right non-dominant side I69033
left dominant side I69032
left non-dominant side I69034

**I69028** **Subarachnoid hemorrhage nontraumatic sequelae Speech/language deficits Other**

Aphasia I69020 Dysphasia I69021
Dysarthria I69022 Fluency disorder I69023

**I609** **Subarachnoid hemorrhage nontraumatic unspecified**

carotid siphon & bifurcation: unspec I6000 right I6001 left I6002
middle cerebral artery: unspec I6010 right I6011 left I6012
anterior communicating artery: I602
posterior communicating artery: unspec I6030 right I6031 left I6032
basilar artery: I604
vertebral artery: unspec I6050 right I6051 left I6052
other intracranial arteries I606
unspecified intracranial artery I607
Other I608

**G44059** **SUNCT: short lasting unilateral neuralgiform headache with conjunctival injection a**

intractable G44051

**K615** **Supralevator abscess**

**I871** **SVCS: superior vena cava syndrome**

**I471** **SVT: supraventricular tachycardia**

**SWALLOWING DIFFICULTY - SEE Dysphagia**

**R55** **Syncope and collapse NOS**

# I10 Cheat Sheet for Home Care - FY 2023

# T

**G44099** **TAC: trigeminal autonomic cephalgia NEC NOS**
intractable G44091

**R000** **Tachycardia NOS**
nonparoxysmal I4589 paroxysmal atrial I471
paroxysmal essential I479 paroxysmal ventricular I472
Postural tachycardia syndrome G90A

**I495** **Tachycardia-bradycardia syndrome**

**R0682** **Tachypnea**

**E8771** **TACO: transfusion associated circulatory overload**

**I71019** **TAD: thoracic aorta dissection unspecified**
ascending aorta I71010 aortic arch I71011
descending thoracic aorta I71012

**B681** **Taenia saginata**

**B680** **Taenia solium intestinal form (cysticercosis)**
larval NOS B699 eye B691
central nervous system B690 myositis B6981
other sites B6989

**719** **Tapeworm NOS**
beef B681 dog B711
pork larva NOS B699 pork NOS B680
fish B700 rat / dwarf B710

**Q262** **TAPVR: total anomalous pulmonary venous return**

**Q872** **TAR: thrombocytopenia w/absent radius syndrome**

**G96191** **Tarlov cyst**

**G5750** **Tarsal tunnel syndrome NOS**
right G5751 left G5752 bilateral G5753

**E7502** **Tay-Sachs disease**

**A159** **TB: tuberculosis respiratory NOS -- SEE Tuberculosis for other sites & sequelae**
respiratory primary A157 lung A150
larynx trachea bronchus A155
intrathoracic lymph nodes A154
other respiratory A158 pleurisy A156

**I495** **TBS: tachycardia bradycardia syndrome**

**J860** **TEF: tracheoesophageal fistula**
following tracheostomy J9504

**M89160** **TEGD: tibial epiphyseal growth disturbance COMPLETE right proximal**
left proximal M89161 right distal M89164 left distal M89165
PARTIAL right proximal M89162
left proximal M89163 right distal M89166 left distal M89167

**M26619** **Temporomandibular joint adhesions & ankylosis unspecified side**

Right M26611 Left M26612 Bilateral M26613

**M26629** **Temporomandibular joint arthralgias unspecified side**

Right M26621 Left M26622 Bilateral M26623

**M26649** **Temporomandibular joint arthritis unspecified**

right M26641 left M26642 bilateral M26643

**M26659** **Temporomandibular joint Arthropathy unspecified**

right M26651 left M26652 bilateral M26653

**M26639** **Temporomandibular joint articular disc disorder unspecified side**

Right M26631 Left M26632 Bilateral M26633

**M26609** **Temporomandibular joint disorder NOS unspecified side**

Right M26601 Left M26602 Bilateral M26603

**M2669** **Temporomandibular joint other disorder**

**Z515** **Terminal care**

**N454** **Testicle abscess**

**E299** **Testicle dysfunction, unspecified**

hypofunction NOS E291 postop hypofunction E895
hyperfunction E290 Other dysfunction E298

**N501** **Testicle hematoma**

**N433** **Testicle hydrocele NOS**

encysted N430 infected N431 other N432

**A5619** **Testicle infection d/t chlamydia trachomatis**

**N50819** **Testicle pain unspecified**

Right N50811 Left N50812

**N500** **Testicular atrophy**

**A35** **Tetanus NOS**

**C710** **Thalamus neoplasm malignant primary**

Secondary C7931 Benign D330
Mets: to bone C7951 to esophageal nodes C771

**G5710** **Thigh lateral cutaneous nerve syndrome unspecified lower limb**

right G5711 left G5712 bilateral G5713

**L97129** **Thigh ulcer non-pressure chronic LEFT NOS**

limited to skin L97121
w/fat layer exposed L97122
w/muscle necrosis L97123
w/bone necrosis L97124
w/muscle involvement w/o necrosis L97125
w/bone involvement w/o necrosis L97126
with other specified severity L97128
CHRONIC RIGHT - Change character #5 to 1
CHRONIC UNSPECIFIED SIDE - Change character #5 to 0

**Thoracic neuritis or radiculitis NOS - SEE Radiculopathy**

**N808** **Thorax endometriosis**

**C140** **Throat neoplasm malignant primary**

Secondary C7989 Benign D109
Mets to bone C7951 mets to esophageal nodes C771
Mets to axilla / arm lymph node C773
Mets to cervical lymph node C770
RELATED: history of tobacco dependence Z87891

**Throat sore SEE SORE THROAT**

**D6949** **Thrombocytopenia primary NOS /other specified**

hereditary & congenital D6942

**D696** **Thrombocytopenia unspecified**

primary NOS D6949 heparin induced SEE HIT
Vaccine-induced / HIT without heparin D7584

**D75839** **Thrombocytosis or Thrombocythemia NOS**

**D75838** **Thrombocytosis Other/Reactive/Secondary**

Code also underlying condition, if known and applicable

**Thrombosis and embolism deep vein NOS arm and leg**

ARM Acute NOS - right I82621 left I82622
bilateral I82623 unspecified I82629
ARM Chronic NOS - right I82721 left I82722
bilateral I82723 unspecified I82729
LEG Acute NOS - right I82401 left I82402
bilateral I82403 unspecified I82409
LEG Chronic NOS - right I82501 left I82502
bilateral I82503 unspecified I82509

**E329** **Thymus disease unspecified**

persistent hyperplasia / hypertrophy E320
aplasia or hypoplasia w/ immunodeficiency D821
abscess E321 other E328

**E060** **Thyroid abscess**

**E034** **Thyroid atrophy acquired**

**THYROID CRISIS OR STORM -- SEE thyrotoxicosis**

**E041** **Thyroid cyst**

**E039** **Thyroid deficit NOS**

d/t iodine / PAS/ iatrogenic E032
postop or d/t radiation therapy E890
congenital E009

**E079** **Thyroid disorder NOS**

enlargement NOS E049
function test abnormal NOS R946
hemorrhage/infarction E0789
infection Echinococcus granulosus B6731
nodule NOS nontoxic E041

**THYROID INSUFFICIENCY -- SEE hypothyroidism**

**E069** **Thyroiditis NOS**

acute/pyogenic E060
chronic NOS / fibrous E065
chronic w/transient thyrotoxicosis E062
autoimmune / Hashimoto's E063
de Quervain's / subacute E061
drug induced E064

**E0590** **Thyrotoxicosis NOS**

w/goiter toxic nodular: NOS E0520 w/crisis E0521
w/goiter uninodular: E0510 w/crisis E0511
w/goiter toxic diffuse: E0500 w/crisis E0501
factitia/ d/t overproduction of TSH: E0540 w/crisis E0541
d/t ectopic thyroid nodule: E0530 w/crisis E0531
NOS w/crisis E0591
RELATED
Cardiomyopathy I43 myopathy G737
Eaton-Lambert Syndrome/ Myasthenia G733

**G459** **TIA: transient ischemic attack**

**F959** **Tic NOS**

drug induced G2561 transient/provisional F950
chronic motor or vocal F951 Tourette's F952
Tic douloureux G500 other of organic origin G2569
other F958

**B359** **Tinea microsporic NOS**

blanca B362 nigra B361 pedis B353
imbricata B355 manuum B352 unguium B351
capitis B350 cruris B356
flava/versicolor B360 corporis B354

**H9319** **Tinnitus NOS unspecified ear**

right ear H9311 left ear H9312 bilateral H9313

**H93A9** **Tinnitus pulsatile unspecified ear**

right H93A1 left H93A2 bilateral H93A3

**TMJ SEE Temporomandibular joint for specific disorders**

**N7093** **TOA: tubo-ovarian abscess NOS salpingitis & oophoritis unspecified**

salpingitis NOS alone N7091
oophoritis NOS alone N7092

**L03039** **Toe cellulitis unspecified**

right L03031 left L03032

**Toe gout ACUTE/NOS (and foot / ankle)**

idiopathic/primary right M10071 left M10072 unsp M10079
lead induced right M10171 left M10172 unsp M10179
drug induced right M10271 left M10272 unsp M10279
d/t renal impairment right M10371 left M10372 unsp M10379
other secondary right M10471 left M10472 unsp M10479

**Toe gout CHRONIC (and foot / ankle)**

idiopathic/primary right M1A071- left M1A072- unsp M1A079-
lead induced right M1A171- left M1A172- unsp M1A179-
drug induced right M1A271- left M1A272- unsp M1A279-
d/t renal impairment right M1A371- left M1A372- unsp M1A379-
other secondary right M1A471- left M1A472- unsp M1A479-
ADD The appropriate 7th character
0 = without tophus (tophi) 1 = with tophus (tophi)

**Toes fracture pathological NOS (Change 4th character to 5 for 'in neoplastic disease')**

unsp M84479- right M84477- left M84478-
7TH character indicates encounter/status
A - initial S - sequela
D - subsequent routine healing
G - subsequent delayed healing
K - subsequent nonunion P - subsequent malunion

**J0390** **Tonsillitis acute NOS**

acute NOS recurrent J0391
strep acute: NOS J0300 recurrent J0301
d/t other spec organism: NOS J0380 recurrent J0381

**M436** **Torticollis NOS**

ocular R29891 hysterical F444
psychogenic F458 spasmodic G243
traumatic recurrent S134

**G540** **TOS: thoracic outlet syndrome**

**M358** **Toxic oil syndrome**

**A483** **Toxic shock syndrome**

**B589** **Toxoplasmosis unspecified**

Toxoplasma oculopathy unspecified B5800
Toxoplasma chorioretinitis B5801
Other toxoplasma oculopathy B5809
Toxoplasma hepatitis B581
Toxoplasma meningoencephalitis B582
Pulmonary toxoplasmosis B583
Toxoplasma myocarditis B5881
Toxoplasma myositis B5882
Toxoplasma tubulo-interstitial nephropathy B5883
Toxoplasmosis with other organ involvement B5889

**C33** **Trachea neoplasm malignant primary**

secondary C7839 benign D142
Mets to bone C7951 mets to unsp lymph nodes C779
Mets to axilla / arm lymph node C773
RELATED
occupational exposure to environmental tobacco smoke Z5731
tobacco use Z720 history of tobacco use Z87891
exposure to environmental tobacco smoke Z7722

**J0410** **Tracheitis acute NOS**

w/obstruction J0411

**Z430** **Tracheostomy care / aftercare**

status w/o need for care Z930

**J9500** **Tracheostomy complication NOS**

stoma hemorrhage J9501 malfunction J9503 other J9509
tracheo-esophageal fistula J9504 stoma infection J9502
For infection code also type of infection: eg. neck cellulitis L038 or a sepsis code

**A719** **Trachoma unspecified**

initial stage A710 active stage A711

**J9584** **TRALI: transfusion related acute lung injury**

**Transfusion reaction hemolytic (blood)**

acute d/t Rh incompatibility T80410- < 24 hrs
acute d/t ABO incompatibility T80310- < 24 hrs
d/t Rh incompatibility T80411- delayed 24 hr+
d/t ABO incompatibility T80311- delayed 24 hr+
d/t Rh incompatibility T80419- unspecified time
d/t ABO incompatibility T80319- unspecified time
7th character indicates encounter
A- initial encounter D- subsequent encounter S- sequela

**Transfusion reaction NON hemolytic (blood)**

ABO incompatibility unsp T8030x-
AB0 incompatibility other spec T8039x-
Rh incompatibility unsp T8040x-
Rh incompatibility other spec T8049x-
7th character indicates encounter
A- initial encounter D- subsequent encounter S- sequela

**M041** **TRAPS: Tumor necrosis factor receptor associated periodic syndrome**

**R251** **Tremor NOS**

essential / familial G250 hysterical F444
intention/ other G252 drug induced G251

**A691** **Trench mouth**

**B75** **Trichinellosis**

**A599** **Trichomoniasis NOS**

intestinal A078 prostatitis A5902
urethritis A5903 urogenital NOS A5900
vulvovaginitis A5901 other specified urogenital A5909
specified site other A598

**I369** **Tricuspid valve disorder nonrheumatic unspecified**

stenosis I360 insufficiency I361
stenosis w/insufficiency I362 other I368

**G509** **Trigeminal nerve disorder NOS**

neuralgia G500 atypical face pain G501

**Trypanosomiasis American SEE Chaga's disease**

**E0580** **TSH: thyroid stimulating hormone overproduction NOS**

with crisis/storm E0581

**A483** **TSS: toxic shock syndrome (also code organism)**

**M3119** **TTP: thrombotic thrombocytopenic purpura**

**A1810** **Tuberculosis genitourinary NOS**

kidney & ureter A1811 bladder A1812
prostate A1814 cervix A1816
vulva A1818 testicles A1816
female pelvic inflammatory disease A1817

**A159** **Tuberculosis respiratory NOS**

respiratory primary A157 lung A150
larynx trachea bronchus A155
ntrathoracic lymph nodes A154
pleurisy A156 other respiratory A158

**B909** **Tuberculosis Sequelae NOS -- Code first the specific condition resulting from TB**

of central nervous system TB B900
of genitourinary TB B901
of bones and joints TB B902
of respiratory and unspecified TB B909 (same as NOS)
of other organs B908

**A219** **Tularemia unspecified**

ulceroglandular A210 oculoglandular A211 pulmonary A212
gastrointestinal A213 generalized A217 other A218

# U

**UCPPS: urologic chronic pelvic pain syndrome No specific code. If term is used, clari**

possible codes
female interstitial cystitis: N3010 w/ hematuria N3011
male chronic prostatitis N411

**UIH: unilateral inguinal hernia SEE Inguinal hernia**

**Ulcer GI peptic SEE Peptic**

**L89899 Ulcer pressure OTHER site unspecified stage (code at site if known)**

unstageable L89890
stage 1 L89891 stage 2 L8992
stage 3 L8993 stage 4 L8994
pressure-induced deep tissue damage L89896

**L8990 Ulcer pressure UNSPECIFIED site unspecified stage(code at site if known)**

unstageable L8995
stage 1 L8991 stage 2 L89892
stage 3 L89893 stage 4 L89894
pressure-induced deep tissue damage L8996

**G5620 Ulnar nerve lesion unspecified upper limb - aka Tardy ulnar nerve palsy**

right G5621 left G5622 bilateral G5623

**N19 Uremia NOS**

chronic N189 extrarenal R392

**Ureter disorders**

adhesions N2889
strangulation/constriction including postop N135
calculus N201 w/calculus of kidney N202
filling defect (found on imaging) R9341
fistula N2889
obstruction due to stone N201
polyp N2889
prolapse NOS N2889 obstructed N135 infected N136

**N80A69 Ureter endometriosis NOS unspecified depth**

Superficial right N80A41 left N80A42 bilateral N80A43 unspecified N80A49
Deep right N80A51 left N80A52 bilateral N80A53 unspecified N80A59
Unspecified depth right N80A61 left N80A62 bilateral N80A63 unspecified N80A69

**T83192- Ureter stent indwelling mechanical complication OTHER**

Mechanical breakdown T83112-
Displacement T83122-
7th character indicates encounter
A- initial encounter D - subsequent encounter S - sequela

**N2886 Ureteritis cystica**

**N2889 Ureterocele**

**N201 Ureteropelvic junction calculus**

**N340** **Urethra abscess**

**N368** **Urethra colic/ cyst/ granuloma**

**N360** **Urethra fistula**

**N3641** **Urethra hypermobility**

**N368** **Urethra instability**

**N3642** **Urethra intrinsic sphincter deficiency**

**N362** **Urethra polyp**

**N368** **Urethra prolapse / rupture nontraumatic**

**N3592** **Urethra stricture FEMALE NOS**

other NEC N3582
post-traumatic d/t childbirth N35021
postop N9912 postinfective NOS N3512

**N35119** **Urethra stricture MALE postinfective NOS**

meatal N35111 bulbous N35112
membranous N35113 anterior N35114
syphilitic A5276 gonococcal A5401

**N99114** **Urethra stricture MALE postop unspecified (includes Postcatheterization)**

meatal N99110 bulbous N99111
membranous N99112 anterior bulbous N991113
fossa navicularis N99115
overlapping sites N99116

**N35014** **Urethra stricture MALE post-traumatic NOS**

meatal N35010 bulbous N35011
membranous N35012 anterior N35013
overlapping sites N35016

**N342** **Urethra ulcer**

**T83091-** **Urethral catheter indwelling mechanical complication OTHER**

displacement T83021- leakage T83031-
mechanical breakdown T83011-
7th character indicates encounter
A- initial encounter D- subsequent encounter S- sequela
SEE cystostomy catheter and nephrostomy catheter at those terms

**T83098-** **Urethral catheter other mechanical complication other**

(includes Hopkins, ileostomy, urostomy catheters)
displacement T83028- leakage T83038-
mechanical breakdown T83018-
7th character indicates encounter
A- initial encounter D- subsequent encounter S- sequela
SEE cystostomy catheter and nephrostomy catheter at those terms

N320 **Urethral contracture/obstruction/stenosis**

R369 **Urethral discharge NOS**

specified w/o blood R360 w/blood R361

N343 **Urethral syndrome unspecified**

N341 **Urethritis infectious nonspecific**

trichomonal A5903 gonococcal A5401
chlamydia trachomatis A5601 candidal B3741

N342 **Urethritis NOS / postmenopausal**

N810 **Urethrocele female**

N360 **Urethrorectal fistula**

R369 **Urethrorrhea NOS**

w/o blood R360 hematospermia R361

N3030 **Urethrotrigonitis NOS**

w/ hematuria N3031

N322 **Urethrovesical fistula**

J069 **URI: upper respiratory infection acute NOS(code infectious agent if known)**

N209 **Urinary calculus NOS**

lower tract specified not bladder N218
lower tract NOS N219 urethra N211
bladder N210 kidney N200
ureter N201 kidney & ureter N202

T83511- **Urinary catheter indwelling infected / inflammed -- Use additional code to identify inf**

7th character indicates encounter
A- initial encounter D- subsequent encounter S- sequela

T83518- **Urinary catheter other infected / inflammed (includes Hopkins catheter, ileostomy, ur**

- Use additional code to identify infection
7th character indicates encounter
A- initial encounter D- subsequent encounter S- sequela

N360 **Urinary fistula NOS**

R32 **Urinary incontinence unspecified**

stress N393 urge N3941
w/o sensory awareness N3942
post-void dribbling N3943 overflow N39490
continuous leakage N3945 postural N39492
mixed urge and stress N3946
functional R3981
RELATED overactive bladder N3281

N390 **Urinary infection NOS (UTI)**

**Urinary tract lower, symptoms SEE LUTS**

**N139** **Urinary tract obstruction NOS**

**R39198** **Urination difficulty other**

hesitancy R3911 weak stream R3912
split stream R3913 urgency R3915
straining R3916 incomplete bladder emptying R3914
need to immediately re-void R39191
position dependent R39192
extravasation of urine R390

**R8289** **Urine abnormal findings on cytological and histological exam other**

pyuria R8281

**R82998** **Urine abnormal findings other (incl cells & casts,crystalluria,melanuria)**

hypocitraturia R82991 hyperuricoscuria R82993
hypercalciuria R82994 hyperoxaluria NOS R82992
hyperoxaluria Primary E7253 Unspecified R8290

**R8279** **Urine culture positive findings**

**R339** **Urine retention NOS**

drug induced R330 psychogenic F458 other R338
RELATED enlarged prostate N401

**M042** **Urticaria familial cold**

**N814** **Uterovaginal prolapse NOS**

complete N813 incomplete N812

**N814** **Uterovaginal prolapse NOS**

Complete N813
Incomplete N812

**N719** **Uterus abscess NOS**

acute/subacute N710 chronic N711

**Z90710** **Uterus absence with cervix absence acquired**

w/ remaining cervical stump acquired Z90711

**N856** **Uterus adhesions/ bands internal**

**N859** **Uterus disorders NOS -- includes ulcer / fibrosis NOS / cyst / atrophy acquired**

endometecified N800 inversion N855
malposition / retroversion M854

**N8000** **Uterus endometriosis unspecified**

Superficial N8001 Deep N8002
Adenomyosis N8003

**Uterus neoplasm**

MALIGNANT primary: NOS C55 isthmus C540
myometrium C542 fundus uteri C543
endometrium C541 overlapping sites C548
corpus uteri unspecified C549
Secondary ANY C7982 Benign ANY D261
Mets to bone C7951 mets to unsp lymph nodes C779
Mets to intrapelvic lymph node C775

**N840** **Uterus polyp NOS**

**N814** **Uterus prolapse NOS --( with vagina prolapse - SEE uterovaginal prolapse)**

**N853** **Uterus subinvolution chronic**

**N390** **UTI: urinary tract infection NOS**

**N139** **UTO: urinary tract obstruction NOS**

# I10 Cheat Sheet for Home Care - FY 2023

**Q872** **VACTERL: vertebrae anus cardiac trachea esophagus renal limbs**

**Z452** **VAD: vascular access device - adjustment & management**

**N895** **Vagina adhesions / atresia NOS**

postop N992

**B3731** **Vagina candidiasis/moniliasis acute -- aka VAGINAL THRUSH, yeast infection**

chronic B3732

**S3023x-** **Vagina contusion**

7th character indicates encounter
A- initial encounter D- subsequent encounter S- sequela

**N898** **Vagina cyst NOS -- includes: of wall / inclusion / squamous cell**

Vagina discharge/leukorrhea NOS same code

**N899** **Vagina disorder unsp noninflammatory**

**N893** **Vagina dysplasia NOS SEE VAIN for intraepithelial neoplasia**

**N8042** **Vagina endometriosis**

**N815** **Vagina enterocele NOS**

**N829** **Vagina fistula NOS**

to small intestine N822 to large intestine N823
to skin / abdominal wall N825 other intetinal tract N824
to bladder N820 other urinary tract N821
other N828

**N898** **Vagina hematoma NOS / hemorrhage NOS**

**A6004** **Vagina herpes simplex**

**R87623** **Vagina high grade squamous intraepithelial lesion from pap smear**

**A5602** **Vagina infection d/t chlamydia trachomatis**

**B3731** **Vagina infection yeast (candidiasis) acute**

chromic B3732

**N898** **Vagina laceration old (includes postop)**

**N894** **Vagina leukoplakia**

**N7681** **Vagina mucositis ulcerative**

RELATED
radiotherapy Y842
antineoplastic drug poisoning:
accidental T451X1- adverse effect T451X5--
undetermined T451X4-
For T codes 7th character indicates encounter
A- initial encounter D- subsequent encounter S- sequela

**C52** **Vagina neoplasm Malignant primary**

Secondary C7982 Benign D281
Mets to bone C7951 mets to unsp lymph nodes C779
Mets to intraabdominal lymph node C772
Mets to intrapelvic lymph node C775

**N842** **Vagina polyp**

**N8189** **Vagina prolapse other w/o uterine prolapse**

with uterus prolapse -- SEE uterovaginal prolapse
of vault after hysterectomy N993
vagina posterior wall prolapse N816
anterior wall: NOS N8110 midline N8111 lateral N8112

**N895** **Vagina stricture / stenosis / atresia**

**N942** **Vaginismus**

psychogenic F525

**N760** **Vaginitis acute / NOS**

chronic / subacute N761
postmenopausal atrophic N952
trichomonal A5901
n other diseases N771
RELATED pinworm B80

**N890** **VAIN: vaginal intraepithelial neoplasia mild grade I**

moderate grade II N891 severe grade III D072

**U070** **Vaping-related disorder**

RELATED
abdominal pain R1084
acute respiratory distress syndrome J80
diarrhea R197
drug-induced interstitial lung disorder J704
lipoid pneumonia J691
weight loss R634

**Varicella SEE Chickenpox**

**I8390** **Varicose veins NOS asymptomatic**

scrotum I861 sublingual I860
pelvis I862 vulva I863 gastric I864
other sites specified NEC I868
SEE leg varicose veins and Esophagus varices for those specified

**Z452** **Vascular access device adjustment and management**

**I7782** **Vasculitis (ANCA): Antineutrophilic cytoplasmic antibody associated**

**R55** **Vasovagal attack**

**Q872** **VATER: vertebrae anus trachea esophagus renal**

**I871** **VCS: vena cava syndrome**

**M5382** **VDTS: video display tube syndrome**

**R403** **Vegetative state persistent**

**T80219-** **Venous central catheter infection unspecified**

bloodstream infection T80211-
local T80212- other T80218-
7th character indicates encounter
A- initial encounter D- subsequent encounter S- sequela

**K432** **Ventral hernia incisional NOS**

incarcerated K430 gangrenous K431

**M4850x-** **Vertebrae collapsed / wedged unsp / non-traumatic compression fx NOS**

occipito-atlanto-axial M4851x-
cervical M4852x- cervicothoracic M4853x-
thoracic M4854x- lumbar M4856x-
thoracolumbar M4855x- lumbosacral M4857x-
sacral and sacrococcygeal M4858x-
7th character indicates encounter:
A= initial encounter
D= subsequent encounter, routine healing
G = subsequent encounter, delayed healing
S = sequela

**M4840x-** **Vertebrae fracture fatigue unspecified**

occipito-atlanto-axial M4841x-
cervical M4842x- cervicothoracic M4843x-
thoracic M4844x- lumbar M4846x-
thoracolumbar M4845x- lumbosacral M4847x-
sacral and sacrococcygeal M4848x-
7th character indicates encounter:
A = initial encounter
D = subsequent encounter, routine healing
G = subsequent encounter, delayed healing
S = sequela

**M1008** **Vertebrae gout acute/NOS -- idiopathic/primary**

lead induced M1018 drug induced M1028
d/t renal impairment M1038 other secondary M1048

**M1A08x-** **Vertebrae gout chronic -- idiopathic/primary**

lead induced M1A18x- drug induced M1A28x-
d/t renal impairment M1A38x- other secondary M1A48x-
ADD the appropriate 7th character
0= without tophus (tophi) 1= with tophus (tophi)

**M2508** **Vertebrae hemarthrosis**

**M8008x-** **Vertebrae osteoporosis age related w/current pathological fracture**

7th character indicates encounter/status
A - initial S - sequela
D - subsequent routine healing
G - subsequent delayed healing
K - subsequent nonunion P - subsequent malunion

**M47029** **Vertebral artery compression syndromes unspecified site**

cervical: M47022
occipito-atlanto-axial: M47021

**I7774** **Vertebral artery dissection**

**I6509** **Vertebral artery occlusion / stenosis NOS unspecified side**

right I6501 left I6502 bilateral I6403

**H8190** **Vertigo (vertiginous) syndrome NOS**

right ear H8191 left ear H8192 bilateral H8193

**H8110** **Vertigo benign positional paroxysmal vertigo NOS**

right ear H8111 left ear H8112 bilateral H8113

**H8109** **Vertigo Meniere's NOS AKA: Meniere's syndrome; labyrinthine hydrops**

right ear H8101 left ear H8102 bilateral H8103

**R42** **Vertigo NOS**

**H81399** **Vertigo peripheral / otogenic NOS AKA Lemoyez' syndrome**

right ear H81391 left ear H81392 bilateral H81393

**N322** **Vesical fistula NEC (excludes fistula to female genital tract)**

**R301** **Vesical tenesmus**

**N321** **Vesicointestinal fistula**

**N1370** **Vesicoureteral reflux unspecified**

specified w/o reflux nephropathy N1371

**Vesicoureteral reflux w/reflux nephropathy**

unilateral N13721 w/hydroureter N13731
bilateral: N13722 w/hydroureter N13732
unspecified: N13729 w/hydroureter N13739

**N820** **Vesicovaginal fistula**

other female urinary-genital fistulae N821

**N900** **VIN: vulvar intraepithelial neoplasia type I mild**

type II N901 type III/severe D071

**A691** **Vincent's gingivitis**

**B3320** **Viral carditis (Coxsackie virus) unspecified**

endocarditis B3321 myocarditis B3322
pericarditis B3323 cardiomyopathy B3324

**B349** **Viremia / viral infection NOS**

**Vitamin deficiency SEE Deficiency (vitamin)**

**H4310** **Vitreous hemorrhage unspecified**

right eye H4311 left eye H4312 bilateral H4313

**E781** **VLDL: very low density lipoid hyperlipoproteinemia**

**R825** **VMA: vanillylmandelic acid elevated in urine**

**T796XX-** **Volkmann's contractures ischemic**

7th character indicates encounter
A- initial encounter D- subsequent encounter S- sequela

**E869** **Volume depletion unspecified**

Dehydration E860
Hypovolemia E861 NOT hypovolemic shock - see shock, hypovolemic
Also code associated disorders of electrolyte and acid-base balance below
Hyperosmolality & hypernatremia (Sodium excess) E870
Hypo-osmolality & hyponatremia (Sodium deficiency) E871
Acidosis E872 Alkalosis E873
Mixed disorder of acid-base balance E874
Hyperkalemia E875 Hypokalemia E876
Electrolyte imbalance NOS E878

**R1110** **Vomiting NOS**

w/o nausea R1111 w/nausea NOS R112
projectile R1112 bilious R1114
fecal matter R1113 hematemesis K920
post-op GI surgery K910
Cyclical: w/migraine G43A0 intractable w/migraine G43A1
Cyclical unrelated to migraine R1115
psychogenic vomiting F5089

**E7401** **von Gierke disease**

**D6800** **Von Willebrand disease, unspecified**

Von Willebrand disease, type 1 D6801
Von Willebrand disease, type 2a D68020
Von Willebrand disease, type 2b D68021
Von Willebrand disease, type 2m D68022
Von Willebrand disease, type 2n D68023
Von Willebrand disease, type 2 unspecified D68029
Von Willebrand disease, type 3 D6803
Von Willebrand disease, acquired D6804
Von Willebrand disease, other D6809

**Z1621** **VRE: vancomycin resistant enterococcus (first code infection)**

**Z1621** **VRSA: vancomycin resistant staph aureus (first code infection)**

**Q210** **VSD: ventricular septal defect congenital**

**N764** **Vulva abscess / furuncle**

**N905** **Vulva atrophy / stenosis**

**B3731** **Vulva candidiasis/moniliasis acute**

chronic B3732

**N907** **Vulva cyst**

**N909** **Vulva disorder unsp noninflammatory**

**N903** **Vulva dysplasia other than VIN Code severe dysplasia as VIN iii**

SEE VIN for intraepithelial dysplasia

**N904** **Vulva dystrophy / kraurosis / leukoplakia**

**N808** **Vulva endometriosis**

**N7682** **Vulva Fournier disease/ gangrene (also vagina)**

**N9089** **Vulva hematoma**

**N9060** **Vulva hypertrophy NOS**

Childhood asymmetric labium majus enlargement N9061
Other specified hypertrophy N9069

**A5602** **Vulva infection d/t chlamydia trachomatis**

**N9089** **Vulva laceration old /scarring**

**N7681** **Vulva mucositis ulcerative**

RELATED
radiotherapy Y842
antineoplastic drug poisoning:
accidental T451X1- adverse effect T451X5-
undetermined T451X4-
For T codes 7th character indicates encounter
A- initial encounter D- subsequent encounter S- sequela

**C519** **Vulva neoplasm MALIGNANT primary unsp / NOS**

labium majus C510 labium minus C511
clitoris C512 overlapping sites C518
SECONDARY C7982 BENIGN D280
Mets to bone C7951 mets to unsp lymph nodes C779
Mets to intraabdominal lymph node C772
Mets to intrapelvic lymph node C775

**N843** **Vulva polyp**

**N9089** **Vulva stricture**

**N766** **Vulva ulcer NOS**

gonococcal infection A5402 syphilis A510
herpesviral [herpes simplex] infection A6004 tuberculosis A1818
in other diseases classified elsewhere N770

**I863** **Vulva varices**

**N94810** **Vulva vestibulitis**

**N942** **Vulvismus**

**N762** **Vulvitis NOS or acute**

subacute / chronic N763

**N94819** **Vulvodynia NOS**

Vulvodynia vestibulitis N94810 other N94818

**N751** **Vulvovaginal gland abscess**

**N760** **Vulvovaginitis NOS / acute**

subacute / chronic N761 candidal/monilial B373
gonococcal A5402 trichomonal B5809
herpetic (simplex) A6004 herpetic (simplex) A6004

**B3731** **VVC: vulvovaginal candidiasis acute**

chronic B3732

**R262** **Walking difficulty NOS**

ataxic gait R260 paralytic gait R261
unsteady on feet R2681 other specified R2689
unspecified gait difficulty R26

**I498** **WAP: wandering atrial pacemaker**

**B079** **Warts viral unspecified**

common B078 plantar B070

**E41** **Wasting d/t malnutrition NOS / extreme**

**G1221** **Wasting d/t paralysis (muscle atrophy)**

**R64** **Wasting disease / syndrome - Code underlying condition first if known**

**M6250** **Wasting of muscles NOS (disuse atrophy NEC**

shoulder: right M62511 left M62512 unsp M62519
upper arm: right M62521 left M62522 unsp M62529
forearm: right M62531 left M62532 unsp M62539
hand: right M62541 left M62542 unsp M62549
thigh: right M62551 left M62552 unsp M62559
lower leg: right M62561 left M62562 unsp M62569
ankle & foot: right M62571 left M62572 unsp M62579
other site M6258 multiple sites NEC M6259

**D72829** **WBC count high NOS**

ymphocytosis D72820 monocytosis D72821
Plasmacytosis D72822 leukemoid reactiion D72823
Basophilia D72824 Bandemia D72825

**D72819** **WBC count low NOS**

lymphocytopenia D72810 other D72818

**R531** **Weakness NOS**

age related R54 Muscle weakness generalized M6281

**A831** **WEE: Western equine encephalitis**

**M3130** **Wegener's granulomatosis/syndrome NOS**

w/renal involvement M3131 other D72828

**R636** **Weight below normal (Code body mass index if known)**

**R635** **Weight gain abnormal**

**R634** **Weight loss abnormal**

**A270** **Weil's disease ( icterohemorrhagica Leptospirosis)**

**E512** **Wernicke's encephalopathy / syndrome**

**A9230** **West Nile Fever NOS**

w/encephalitis A9231
w/neuro complication except encephalitis A9232
w/complication other than neuro A9239

**Z993** **Wheelchair dependence Code cause first**

**Z4689** **Wheelchair fitting & adjustment**

**R062** **Wheezing -- do not code with asthma**

**B362** **White piedra**

**WNF: SEE West Nile Fever**

**A4852** **Wound botulism**

**Wound care**

change/remove dsg nonsurgical/NOS wound Z480
change/remove dsg surgical wound Z4801
remove sutures or staples Z4802
change/remove drain Z4803

**Wound dehiscence**

wound disruption NOS T8130x-
surgical wound skin & subcut tissue disruption T8131x-
surgical wound deep / internal disruption T8132x-
of traumatic injury wound repair T8133x-
For above codes, 7th character indicates encounter
A- initial encounter D- subsequent encounter S- sequela
amputation stump disruption T8781

**Z4803** **Wound drain postop change / removal**

**T8140x-** **Wound infection postop NEC any site except OB**

superficial incisional surgical site T8141x-
deep incisional surgical site T8142x-
organ and space surgical site T8143x-
other surgical site T8149x-
Sepsis following a procedure T8144x-
7th character indicates encounter
A- initial encounter D- subsequent encounter S- sequela

**T8184X-** **Wound surgical non-healing**

7th character indicates encounter
A- initial encounter D- subsequent encounter S- sequela

**T798XX-** **Wound traumatic slow/non healing**

7th character indicates encounter
A- initial encounter D- subsequent encounter S- sequela

**I456** **WPW: Wolff Parkinson White syndrome**

**M25739** **Wrist bone spur (osteophyte) unspecified**

right M25731 left M25732

**M71439** **Wrist calcification unspecified**

right M71431 left M71432

**M94239** **Wrist chondromalacia unspecified**

right M94231 left M94232

**M21339** **Wrist drop acquired unspecified side**

right M21331 left M21332

**S62109-** **Wrist fracture NOS**

right wrist unspecified carpal bone S62101-
left wrist unspecified carpal bone S62102-
Add the appropriate 7th character:
A- initial encounter for closed fracture
B - initial encounter for open fracture
D - subsequent encounter for fracture with routine healing
G - subsequent encounter for fracture with delayed healing
K - subsequent encounter for fracture with nonunion
P - subsequent encounter for fracture with malunion
S - sequela

**Wrist gout acute/NOS**

idiopathic/primary right M10031 left M10032 unsp M10039
lead induced right M10131 left M10132 unsp M10139
drug induced right M10231 left M10232 unsp M10239
d/t renal impairment right M10331 left M10332 unsp M10339
other secondary right M10431 left M10432 unsp M10439

**Wrist gout chronic**

idiopathic/primary right M1A031- left M1A032- unsp M1A039-
lead induced right M1A131- left M1A132- unsp M1A139-
drug induced right M1A231- left M1A232- unsp M1A239-
d/t renal impairment right M1A331- left M1A332- unsp M1A339-
Other secondary right M1A431- left M1A432- unsp M1A439-
ADD the appropriate 7th character
0 = without tophus (tophi) 1 = with tophus (tophi)

**M25039** **Wrist hemarthrosis unspecified**

right M25031 left M25032

**M25539** **Wrist pain NOS unspecified**

right M25531 left M25532

**R238** **Xanthosis**

**A669** **Yaws unspecified**

Latent A668
Bone and joint lesions A666
Gangosa A665
Gummata and ulcers A664
Hyperkeratosis A663
Multiple papillomata and wet crab yaws A661
Other early skin lesions A662
Initial lesions A660

**A925** **Zika virus disease**

congenital P354
Contact with and (suspected) exposure to Z20821
Includes conditions recorded as fever, infection, NOS
RELATED Microcephaly Q02

**Zona - SEE Herpes Zoster**

# TABLES

**Aftercare**

**Medication Long-term Use**

**Ulcers, External**
**Pressure & Non-pressure with Related Conditions**

# Aftercare, Patient care, Caregiver Training

Z4682  Catheter non-vascular  fitting and adjustment
Z452    Catheter vascular adjustment and management

**Counseling**
Alcohol abuse counseling and surveillance of alcoholic  Z7141
Alcohol abuse counseling for family member of alcoholic  Z142
Dietary counseling and surveillance   Z713
Drug abuse counseling and surveillance of drug abuser   Z7151
Drug abuse counseling for family member of abuser  Z7152
Exercise counseling   Z71.82
Test findings explained    Z712
Fear of health concern without diagnosis  Z711
Human immunodeficiency virus [HIV] counseling    Z717
Immunization safety counseling  Z7185
    Code also, if applicable,
    Encounter for immunization Z23
    Immunization not carried out due to patient having had the disease Z2881
    Immunization not carried out because of caregiver refusal  Z2882
    Immunization not carried out due to unavailability of vaccine Z2883
    Immunization not carried out for other reason  Z2889
    Immunization not carried out for unspecified reason  Z289
Medical advice NOS, other unspecified counseling Z719
Spiritual or religious counseling  Z7181
Third party counseling on behalf of absent regarding advice or treatment of client/patient Z710
Tobacco abuse counseling   Z716

**Digestive tract**
Colostomy complication, unspecified K9400
Colostomy complications other of colostomy  K9409
Colostomy encounter for attention to   Z433
Colostomy granulation of surrounding skin   L929
Colostomy hemorrhage K9401
Colostomy infection K9402
Colostomy malfunction /Mechanical complication K9403
Colostomy status only, without need for care  Z933
Enterostomy complication, unspecified K9410
Enterostomy hemorrhage K9411
Enterostomy infection K9412
Enterostomy malfunction / mechanical complication  K9413
Enterostomy other complications of  K9419
Enterostomy status only, without need for care Z934
Esophagostomy complications, unspecified  K9430
Esophagostomy hemorrhage  K9431
Esophagostomy infection K9432    Use additional code to identify the infection
Esophagostomy malfunction/mechanical complication  K9433
Gastric lap band encounter for fitting and adjustment  Z4651
Other complications of esophagostomy  K9439

Gastrostomy status only, without need for care Z931
Gastrostomy encounter for attention to Z431
Gastrostomy complication, unspecified K9420
Gastrostomy hemorrhage K9421
Gastrostomy infection K9422 Use additional code to specify type of infection
Gastrostomy malfunction / mechanical complication of gastrostomy K9423
Other complications of gastrostomy K9429
Ileostomy status only, without need for care Z932
Ileostomy encounter for attention to Z432

Encounter for fitting and adjustment of gastric lap band
Encounter for fitting and adjustment of other gastrointestinal appliance and device Z4659
Encounter for attention to other artificial openings of digestive tract Z434
Cellulitis of abdominal wall L03311

## **Drug level monitoring encounter for** Z5181
Z451 Infusion pump adjustment and management
Z46.81 Insulin pump fitting & adjustment, titration, instruction & training

## Orthopedic aftercare
Z4732 Following explantation of hip joint prosthesis
Z4731 Following explantation of shoulder joint prosthesis
Z4733 Aftercare following explantation of knee joint prosthesis
Z471 Following joint replacement surgery
**Use additional** code from the presence table below to identify the joint
Z4782 Encounter for orthopedic aftercare following scoliosis surgery
Z4781 Encounter for orthopedic aftercare following surgical amputation
Z4789 Encounter for other orthopedic aftercare

**Presence of orthopedic joint replacement**

| | Right | Left | Unspecified | Bilateral |
|---|---|---|---|---|
| Shoulder | **Z96611** | **Z96612** | **Z966119** | |
| Elbow | **Z96621** | **Z96622** | **Z96629** | |
| Wrist | **Z96631** | **Z96632** | **Z96639** | |
| Hip | **Z96641** | **Z96642** | **Z96649** | **Z96643** |
| Knee | **Z96651** | **Z96652** | **Z96659** | **Z96653** |
| Ankle | **Z96661** | **Z96662** | **Z96669** | |
| Finger | **Z96691** | **Z96692** | | **Z96693** |
| Unspecified | **Z9660** | | | |
| Other | **Z96698** | | | |

Z5189 Other specified aftercare
Z4689 Other specified devices fitting & adjustment
Z515 Palliative care
Z5189 Physical therapy

**Postop Aftercare**, following surgery on
Circulatory system Z48812
Digestive system Z48815
Genitourinary system Z48816
sterilization reversal Z3142
Neoplasm Z483
Use additional code to identify the neoplasm
Nervous system Z48811
sense organs Z48810
Oral cavity / teeth Z48814
Other specified surgical aftercare Z4889
Respiratory system Z48813
Skin and subcutaneous tissue Z48817

**Screening, Encounter for**
Human immunodeficiency virus [HIV] Z114
Human papillomavirus (HPV) Z1151
Tuberculosis Respiratory Z111
Tuberculosis latent Z117
Infections with a predominantly sexual mode of transmission Z113

**Tracheostomy**
Tracheostomy status only, without need for care Z930
Tracheostomy encounter for attention to Z430
Tracheostomy complication unspecified J9500
Tracheostomy stoma hemorrhage from J9501
Tracheostomy stoma infection of J9502
Tracheostomy cause of tracheal stenosis / mechanical complication J9503
Tracheostomy related tracheo-esophageal fistula J9504
Tracheostomy other complication J9509
Cellulitis of neck L038

**Urinary Tract**
Unspecified cystostomy status Z9350
Cutaneous-vesicostomy status Z9351
Appendico-vesicostomy status Z9352
Other cystostomy status Z9359
Other artificial openings of urinary tract status Z936
Cystostomy encounter for attention to Z435
Cystostomy hemorrhage N99510
Cystostomy infection N99511
Cystostomy malfunction N99512
Other cystostomy complication N99518
Cystostomy catheter, leakage of T83030-
Cystostomy mechanical complication T83090- (other / mechanical obstruction / perforation /protrusion )
Cystostomy displacement T83020-
Cystostomy breakdown (mechanical) T83010-
For 'T' codes above add appropriate 7th character:
A=initial encounter D-subsequent encounter S=sequela
Nephrostomy attention to Z436
Z4901 Renal dialysis catheter extracorporeal encounter for fitting and adjustment/removal/replacement / toilet/cleansing
Ureterostomy or urethrostomy attention to Z436
Urinary tract other artificial openings attention to (not elsewhere in this list) Z436

Z437  Vagina artificial attention to
Z452   Vascular access device adjustment and management

Z4689 Wheelchair fitting & adjustment

**Wound Care** non-traumatic (for aftercare following injury, code injury, by site, with 7th character for subsequent encounter)
Z4800  Change or remove non-surgical wound dressing
(wound dressing NOS)
Z4803 Change or remove drains
Z4801 Change or remove surgical wound dressing
Z4802  Remove staples or sutures

Z43.9  Unspecified artificial opening attention to
Z469   Unspecified device fitting & adjustment

# Medications long term current use

| |
|---|
| Alkylating agent Z79630 |
| Analgesic opiate / use of methadone for pain management Z79891 |
| Antibiotics Z792 |
| Anticoagulants Z7901 |
| Antimetabolite agent Z79631 |
| Antithrombotics/antiplatelets Z7902 |
| Antitumor antibiotic Z79632 |
| |
| Aspirin Z7982 |
| Bisphosphonates Z7983 |
| Calcineurin inhibitor Z79621 |
| Estrogen selective receptors modulators (SERMs) (raloxifene, tamoxifen, toremifene) Z79810<br>aromatase inhibitors (anastrozole, exemestane, letrozole) Z79811<br>other agents affecting (down regulators) Z79818 |
| Hormonal contraceptives / use of birth control pill or patch Z793 |
| Hormone replacement therapy (postmenopausal) Z79890 |
| Hypoglycemic oral drugs Z7984 |
| Hypoglycemic injectables Z7985 |
| Immunosuppressive biologic Z79620 |
| Insulin Z794 |
| Mitotic inhibitor Z79633 |
| MTOR inhibitor Z79623 |
| Myelosuppressive agent Z7964 |
| Non-steroidal anti-inflammatories (NSAID) Z791 |
| Nucleotide synthesis inhibitor Z79624 |
| Other long term (current) drug therapy Z79899 |
| Steroids long term (current) use, inhaled Z7951<br>Steroids long term (current) use, systemic Z7952 |
| Topoisomerase inhibitor Z79634 |

# ULCERS, EXTERNAL

When applicable, first code varicose ulcers, associated gangrene, atherosclerosis of the lower extremities, chronic venous hypertension, diabetic ulcers, postphlebitic syndrome, postthrombotic syndrome given on following pages.

## Non-pressure chronic ulcer of lower limb

| | Thigh | Calf | Ankle | Heel & Midfoot | Other part of foot /toe | Other part of lower leg | Unspec part of lower leg |
|---|---|---|---|---|---|---|---|
| Skin Breakdown | Right **L97111**<br>Left **L97121**<br>Unsp **L97101** | Right **L97211**<br>Left **L97221**<br>Unsp **L97201** | Right **L97311**<br>Left **L97321**<br>Unsp **L97301** | Right **L97411**<br>Left **L97421**<br>Unsp **L97401** | Right **L97511**<br>Left **L97521**<br>Unsp **L97501** | Right **L97811**<br>Left **L97821**<br>Unsp **L97801** | Right **L97911**<br>Left **L97921**<br>Unsp **L97901** |
| **fat layer exposed** | Right **L97112**<br>Left **L97122**<br>Unsp **L97102** | Right **L97212**<br>Left **L97222**<br>Unsp **L97202** | Right **L97312**<br>Left **L97322**<br>Unsp **L97302** | Right **L97412**<br>Left **L97422**<br>Unsp **L97402** | Right **L97512**<br>Left **L97522**<br>Unsp **L97502** | Right **L97812**<br>Left **L97822**<br>Unsp **L97802** | Right **L97912**<br>Left **L97922**<br>Unsp **L97902** |
| **Muscle necrosis** | Right L**97113**<br>Left **L97123**<br>Unsp **L97103** | Right **L97213**<br>Left **L97223**<br>Unsp **L97203** | Right **L97313**<br>Left **L97323**<br>Unsp **L97303** | Right **L97413**<br>Left **L97423**<br>Unsp **L97403** | Right **L97513**<br>Left **L97523**<br>Unsp **L97503** | Right **L97813**<br>Left **L97823**<br>Unsp **L97803** | Right **L97913**<br>Left **L97923**<br>Unsp **L97903** |
| Bone Necrosis | Right L**97114**<br>Left **L97124**<br>Unsp **L97104** | Right **L97214**<br>Left **L97224**<br>Unsp **L97204** | Right **L97314**<br>Left **L97324**<br>Unsp **L97304** | Right **L97414**<br>Left **L97424**<br>Unsp **L97404** | Right **L97514**<br>Left **L97524**<br>Unsp **L97504** | Right **L97814**<br>Left **L97824**<br>Unsp **L97804** | Right **L97914**<br>Left **L97924**<br>Unsp **L97904** |
| Muscle w/o necrosis | Right **97115**<br>Left **L97125**<br>Unsp **L97105** | Right **L97215**<br>Left **L97225**<br>Unsp **L97205** | Right **L97315**<br>Left **L97325**<br>Unsp **L97305** | Right **L97415**<br>Left **L97425**<br>Unsp **L97405** | Right **L97515**<br>Left **L97525**<br>Unsp **L97505** | Right **L97815**<br>Left **L97825**<br>Unsp **L97805** | Right **L97915**<br>Left **L97925**<br>Unsp **L97905** |
| Bone w/o necrosis | Right L**97116**<br>Left **L97126**<br>Unsp **L97106** | Right **L97216**<br>Left **L97226**<br>Unsp **L97206** | Right **L97316**<br>Left **L97326**<br>Unsp **L97306** | Right **L97416**<br>Left **L97426**<br>Unsp **L97406** | Right **L97516**<br>Left **L97526**<br>Unsp **L97506** | Right **L97816**<br>Left **L97826**<br>Unsp **L97806** | Right **L97916**<br>Left **L97926**<br>Unsp **L97906** |
| Other specified | Right L**97118**<br>Left **L97128**<br>Unsp **L97108** | Right **L97218**<br>Left **L97228**<br>Unsp **L97208** | Right **L97318**<br>Left **L97328**<br>Unsp **L97308** | Right **L97418**<br>Left **L97428**<br>Unsp **L97408** | Right **L97518**<br>Left **L97528**<br>Unsp **L97508** | Right **L97818**<br>Left **L97828**<br>Unsp **L97808** | Right **L97918**<br>Left **L97928**<br>Unsp **L97908** |
| Unspecified | Right L**97119**<br>Left **L97129**<br>Unsp **L97109** | Right **L97219**<br>Left **L97229**<br>Unsp **L97209** | Right **L97319**<br>Left **L97329**<br>Unsp **L97309** | Right **L97419**<br>Left **L97429**<br>Unsp **L97409** | Right **L97519**<br>Left **L97529**<br>Unsp **L97509** | Right **L97819**<br>Left **L97829**<br>Unsp **L97809** | Right **L97919**<br>Left **L97929**<br>Unsp **L97909** |

## Other Non-pressure chronic ulcers

**Buttock** L9841-
**Back** L9842-
**Skin of other sites** L9849-

Replace dash in codes at left to specify degree of involvement
1=limited to breakdown of skin
2=with fat layer exposed
3=with necrosis of muscle
4=necrosis of bone
9=with unspecified severity

## Pressure ulcers

| | |
|---|---|
| Elbow unspecified L8900-<br>right L8901-<br>left L8902- | Use list below to replace dash to specify severity<br><br>Unstageable = 0<br>stage 1 = 1<br>stage 2 = 2<br>stage 3 = 3<br>stage 4 = 4<br>unspecified stage = 9<br>pressure-induced deep-tissue damage = 6 |
| Back unspecified part L8910-<br>right upper L8911-<br>left upper L8912-<br>right lower L8913-<br>left lower L8914- | |
| Sacral region L8915- | |
| Hip unspecified L8920<br>right hip L8921-<br>left hip L8922- | |
| Buttock unspecified L8930-<br>right buttock L8931-<br>left buttock L8932- | |
| Contiguous site of back, buttock and hip L894- | |
| Ankle unspecified L8950-<br>right ankle L8951-<br>left ankle L8952- | |
| Heel unspecified L8960-<br>right heel L8961-<br>left heel L8962- | |
| Head L8981- | |
| Other site L8989- | |
| Unspecified site L899- | |

| Varicose veins lower extremities w/ulcer, with or w/o inflammation | | | |
|---|---|---|---|
| | Right with ulcer | Left with ulcer | Unspecified with ulcer |
| Thigh | I83011 | I83021 | I83001 |
| Calf | I83012 | I83022 | I83002 |
| Ankle | I83013 | I83023 | I83003 |
| Heel & midfoot | I83014 | I83024 | I83004 |
| Other part of foot | I83015 | I83025 | I83005 |
| Other part lower leg | I83018 | I83028 | I83008 |
| Unspecified site | I83019 | I83029 | I83009 |
| | Right with ulcer & inflammation | Left with ulcer & inflammation | Unspecified with ulcer & inflammation |
| Thigh | I83211 | I83221 | I83201 |
| Calf | I83212 | I83222 | I83202 |
| Ankle | I83213 | I83223 | I83203 |
| Heel & midfoot | I83214 | I83224 | I83204 |
| Other part of foot | I83215 | I83225 | I83205 |
| Other part lower leg | I83218 | I83228 | I83208 |
| Unspecified site | I83219 | I83229 | I83209 |
| **Varicose veins lower extremities w/inflammation only** | | | |
| Varicose veins of unspecified lower extremity with inflammation I8310 | | | |
| Varicose veins of right lower extremity with inflammation I8311 | | | |
| Varicose veins of left lower extremity with inflammation I8312 | | | |
| | | | |
| **Varicose veins of leg with pain or other complications** | | | |
| | with pain | W/ other complications | Asymptomatic |
| Right | I83811 | I83891 | I8391 |
| Left | I83812 | I83892 | I8392 |
| Bilateral | I83813 | I83893 | I8393 |
| Unspecified | I83819 | I83899 | I8390 |
| | | | |

## **Asymptomatic** varicose veins of lower extremities

**Unspecified / Varicose veins NOS I8390**
**right lower extremity I8391**
**left lower extremity I8392**
**bilateral lower extremities I8393**

| **Diabetic ulcers** - Code before chronic or pressure ulcers | |
|---|---|
| Diabetes mellitus due to underlying condition with foot ulcer E08621 | Diabetes mellitus due to underlying condition with other skin ulcer E08622 |
| Drug or chemical induced diabetes mellitus with foot ulcer E09621 | Drug or chemical induced diabetes mellitus with other skin ulcer E09622 |
| Type 1 diabetes mellitus with foot ulcer E10621 | Type 1 diabetes mellitus with other skin ulcer E10622 |
| Type 2 diabetes mellitus with foot ulcer E11621 | Type 2 diabetes mellitus with other skin ulcer E11622 |
| Other specified diabetes mellitus with foot ulcer E13621 | Other specified diabetes mellitus with other skin ulcer E13622 |

## Other Related Codes

| **Gangrene**, not elsewhere classified / Gangrenous cellulitis I96 | | | | |
|---|---|---|---|---|
| | | | | |
| **Lower extremity** Chronic **venous hypertension** (idiopathic) | Right | Left | Bilateral | Unspecified |
| with ulcer | I87311 | I87312 | I87313 | I87319 |
| with ulcer and inflammation | I87331 | I87332 | I87333 | I87339 |
| | | | | |
| **Postphlebitic / postthrombotic syndrome of lower extremity** | | | | |
| | Right | Left | Bilateral | Unspecified |
| with ulcer | I87011 | I87012 | I87013 | I87019 |
| with ulcer and inflammation | I87031 | I87032 | I87033 | I87039 |

Made in United States
North Haven, CT
05 November 2026

21766932R00122